D1383019

Stress and Distress among the Unemployed
Hard Times and Vulnerable People

PLENUM STUDIES IN WORK AND INDUSTRY

Series Editors:
Ivar Berg, *University of Pennsylvania, Philadelphia, Pennsylvania*
and Arne L. Kalleberg, *University of North Carolina, Chapel Hill, North Carolina*

WORK AND INDUSTRY
Structures, Markets, and Processes
Arne L. Kalleberg and Ivar Berg

Current Volumes in the Series:

ANALYZING THE LABOR FORCE
Concepts, Measures, and Trends
Clifford C. Clogg, Scott R. Eliason, and Kevin T. Leicht

EMPLOYMENT RELATIONS IN FRANCE
Evolution and Innovation
Alan Jenkins

ENDING A CAREER IN THE AUTO INDUSTRY
"30 and Out"
Melissa A. Hardy, Lawrence Hazelrigg, and Jill Quadagno

NEGRO BUSINESS AND BUSINESS EDUCATION
Their Present and Prospective Development
Joseph A. Pierce
Introduction by John Sibley Butler

THE OPERATION OF INTERNAL LABOR MARKETS
Staffing Practices and Vacancy Chains
Lawrence T. Pinfield

SEGMENTED LABOR, FRACTURED POLITICS
Labor Politics in American Life
William Form

THE SOCIAL AND SPATIAL ECOLOGY OF WORK
The Case of a Survey Research Organization
Rita Gorawara-Bhat

SOURCEBOOK OF LABOR MARKETS
Evolving Structures and Processes
Edited by Ivar Berg and Arne L. Kalleberg

STRESS AND DISTRESS AMONG THE UNEMPLOYED
Hard Times and Vulnerable People
Clifford L. Broman, V. Lee Hamilton, and William S. Hoffman

A Chronological Listing of Volumes in this series appears at the back of this volume.

A Continuation Order Plan is available for this series. A continuation order will bring delivery of each new volume immediately upon publication. Volumes are billed only upon actual shipment. For further information please contact the publisher.

Stress and Distress among the Unemployed

Hard Times and Vulnerable People

Clifford L. Broman

Michigan State University
East Lansing, Michigan

V. Lee Hamilton

University of Maryland
College Park, Maryland

and

William S. Hoffman

International Union—UAW (Retired)
Detroit, Michigan

Kluwer Academic / Plenum Publishers
New York · Boston · Dordrecht · London · Moscow

Library of Congress Cataloging-in-Publication Data

Broman, Clifford L.
    Stress and distress among the unemployed: hard times and vulnerable people/Clifford
L. Broman, V. Lee Hamilton, William S. Hoffman.
        p.   cm. — (Plenum studies in work and industry)
    Includes bibliographical references and index
    ISBN 0-306-46329-6
        1. Unemployment—Psychological aspects.   2. Unemployed—Psychology.   3.   Stress
(Psychology)   I. Hamilton, V. Lee.   II. Hoffman, William Sydney, 1944–   III. Title.   IV.
Series.

HD5708 .B76 2000
331.13'7'019—dc21

                                                                                                00-022847

ISBN: 0-306-46329-6

©2001 Kluwer Academic / Plenum Publishers
233 Spring Street, New York, N.Y. 10013

http://www.wkap.nl/

10 9 8 7 6 5 4 3 2 1

A C.I.P. record for this book is available from the Library of Congress

Printed in the United States of America

To my family

Preface

The 1987 General Motors plant closings represented a major upheaval for thousands of workers, for the union that represented those workers, and for the communities they called home. This book tells the story of what happened to workers affected by these plant closings. More generally, it deals with the stress of job loss and with possible ways of coping with that stress.

We wish this book were out of date. We wish that the phenomenon of which it speaks—plant closings and their human consequences—had ceased to be. Instead, the book chronicles what was, at the time, the largest series of plant closings by a single employer—General Motors' 1987 plant closings—but it does so in the shadow of a much larger set of closings by that same employer that occurred later. "Our" closings promised job losses of 29,000, largely concentrated in the rust belt of Michigan and its environs. The next round of closings period hit many more GM workers nationwide in the 1992–1995 period. GM's original announcement of the new closings in February of 1992 promised 21 plants would be shut, 74,000 jobs eliminated, and the Board of Directors planned to eliminate a total of 120,000 jobs during the 1990s. (*Time*, November 9, 1992, pp. 43–44).

Such events attract intense interest across the social sciences. A massive wave of plant closings can attract the attention of economists, historians, sociologists, psychologists, anthropologists, and political scientists. Therefore it is important at the outset to make clear what our focus and our claims will be. We cannot grasp the entire whole of plant closings and their economic, social, and political consequences. Our study has a more micro–level focus. It looks at blue collar work and union membership through the eyes of individual workers interviewed before and after the plants closed in 1987. The goal is to paint a social psychology of the despair of job loss, workers' hopes for the future, and how workers turn despair into hope.

Researchers have been examining the factors and forces which precipitate plant closings for decades. The literal aging of a nation's industrial capacity obviously contributes to plant closings. But this is not the critical issue. If plants that get old were simply closed and replaced, nearby, with a new plant there would be no cause for concern among the workers or anybody else. But what is happening is that plants—some old, some middle–aged, some not–so–old–at–all—are being closed and nothing is springing up in their place.   How does this come to be? Among the explanations scholars have come up with are such factors as labor costs, avoidance of unions, capital flight to cheaper markets, foreign competition and the like. In keeping with our desire to paint a social psychology of the workers affected by plant closings, we wondered what the workers' own theories were. How did they come to terms with why their plants were closing? And what did they think would come of it?

The question about "who or what is responsible for your job situation" was answered, by most workers, as if the question had been, "Who caused the plant to close?"   The following seven statements illustrate how workers tended to interweave thoughts about GM, general economic factors, and such particulars as the role of government or of free trade agreements:

1. "General Motors wanted to close the plants because they can make a better return on their investments outside the country."
2. "The sagging market for American cars is because of imports. The other big reason was outsourcing for parts we used to make here."
3. "The government is letting jobs go out to the cheaper overseas markets and they are shipping the jobs out of Michigan for cheaper labor."
4. "GM plans to be more competitive with the Japanese. To do this they discontinue our jobs and outsource parts so they don't have to pay high wages to union workers."
5. "It is Reagan's fault. He lifted the import restrictions and the imports just came pouring in."
6. "They could have stayed in Michigan and condensed the plants in the area. But, GM is looking for cheaper labor and places to operate that are more economical for their profits."
7. "GM wanted more profits—with no consideration for the working man. They could make cars cheaper somewhere else so they shut down our plant."

These were workers with first–hand experience inside the plants. They had little or no exposure to the research literature about plant closings and job loss. The language they use is simple and straightforward. Their attitudes are more visceral than intellectualized. Yet their image of the subject matter was consonant with the conclusions of many academic critics about what is producing the phenomenon we call plant closings.

There is a common theme running through these opinions. Many workers seem to see plant closings, free trade agreements, and outsourcing as a combined assault on organized labor in the United States. They believe that the logic of profit accumulation has led General Motors to use plant closings to try to break the back of organized labor and to undercut the cost of a decent living for working men and women. They see the movement toward a global economy as an attempt by auto manufacturers to abandon a mature industrialized labor force (which costs them more money) and to replace it with more docile workers from cheaper and unorganized international markets.

Whether they are right or wrong is not the issue. This is what they saw, circa 1987, just before the plants shut down. This is the crisis—in the language of social science, the "stressor"— with which they had to cope.

This book tells a story of losses. When workers' jobs are lost, or even threatened, they pay an economic and emotional price. Their financial security is shaken. Their home life is racked by strife between parent and child and between partner and partner. And their peace of mind—their sense of balance between the stresses of life and their ability to cope with those stresses—is disturbed.

This book also tells a story of strengths. We argue that it is part of the human condition to be susceptible to distress—to depression and anxiety, despair and fear—when objective circumstances are bad enough. We will seek both the causes and the cures of these workers' woes in the economic and social cards life deals them.

One message which emerges is that life is a stacked deck. Certain workers are better prepared to cope with the financial troubles that accompany a plant closing than others. Some have more money to start with, like high income workers. Some have more of a chance to regain jobs, or feel they do, like better educated or high seniority workers. Certain workers are likely to be facing more troubles in life anyway—whether or not a plant closes. And if these workers just happen to find themselves more often in an closing plant, life has just hit them with a double whammy. As later chapters will outline, some workers had it relatively easy or brutally rough simply because of who they were, or who they were *in combination with* where they were (in a closing plant, and then unemployed).

One of the things that gives people reason to believe is what they can see in themselves: what resources they have, what drawbacks they will acknowledge, what past they can draw on for comfort and what future they can envision for hope. In later chapters, we also look into workers' thoughts and feelings about themselves and their lives. Here we find certain psychological strengths, such as the ability to cope with the situation in a way that offers hope and some semblance of a sense of control over fate. Within limits, what people believe to be true shapes what is true.

Other reasons to believe come from the world around us, from our intimate and not–so–intimate social ties. People don't solve the great crises of life alone, no matter what their collection of badges of status and worth. Blue collar workers are no exception. Workers have several traditional means of coping with tragedy. One is religion, a cry for help directed upward. Another is loved ones and friends, the sort of help that can be found around one's own back yard. Yet another is a labor organization. Each of these means is in some sense collective, whether it refers to the bonds of a religious community, the arms of those who care about us most, or the brother–and–sisterhood of those who share our way of making a living in this world. Other ways of getting help such as seeing a mental health professional, in contrast, focus on the individual who is in trouble. But when plants close down, the trouble that ensues is collective trouble.

When a crisis strikes we need all the help we can get. Our concluding arguments will focus on the necessity of combating the impact of plant closings through multiple factors, but especially the collective forces our workers drew upon for strength. When woes are spread across a plant, or a state, or a nation, many forces come together to explain the resilience of those workers who survive the crisis and the despair of the rest. What gives hope is an amalgam, a combination, of reasons to believe in the self and the future. Much of the help is collective. It is drawn from other people and groups rather than from some hardy self–reliant psychological interior. Hope may spring eternal in the human breast, but other people help to put it there and to nurture it. Help comes to workers from those they love, from a God they worship actively, and from the union to which they belong.

In summary, this is a study of unemployment and mental health, but it is also a study of coping and survival. Because as much as we want to know what happens to people and their families when jobs are lost, we are also critically interested in what they do to survive the hard times. We will see both in this book; who lost jobs and why, how people tried to cope with the situation, and importantly, that the resilience of the human spirit kept people going through the hard times. While this is a book about loss, it is also a book about how people move on from loss. The book is a tribute to the men and women of the UAW; we celebrate their resilience and courage in the face of loss.

Funds for the research were provided by the Michigan Health Care Research and Education Foundation, (now the Blue Cross Blue Shield Foundation of Michigan) and by the International Union–UAW. We are especially grateful to the men and women of the UAW, whose experiences and views form this investigation.

We also acknowledge the patience and encouragement of our families, for putting up with us while we were writing this book. They, too, are a resilient bunch.

Contents

Chapter 6

Chapter 7

Chapter 8

Psychological Resources and Distress 161

Chapter 9

Individual versus Collective Resources 185

Chapter 10

Conclusions: What Have We Learned?.. 211

1

Introduction: Stress and the Life Course during Hard Times

My elders used to tell me that you get in there and get some time in and you're set for life. They said you'd never have to worry about a job once you're in with GM. But that's not how it turned out to be. The way things are going, someday soon the only ones left working for them will be technicians and robot repair people. They won't even need all the fancy management anymore. My kids will never work in a factory. I tell them to get an education—get into computers or something. No, it's all over. And what call for labor they will have comes from Mexico or Asia or someplace.

—a closing plant worker

You have to know what it is like. We got the quality up. We did our share and more. They just closed us anyway. You hear about how we just didn't care about the place or anything. We really did care and we cared about each other too. Nobody wanted this and we all pulled together to make it work. No one wants to just get laid off and end up grubbing. We were motivated. We exceeded even the company's expectations. So why? All I know is that when you bust your ass and get kicked in the head anyway, it does something to you. You get depressed. In the end we were all depressed.

—a closing plant worker

The 1987 General Motors plant closings represented a major upheaval for thousands of workers, for the union that represented those workers, and for the communities they called home. This book tells the story of what happened to workers affected by these plant closings. More generally, it deals with the stress of job loss and with possible ways of coping with that stress.

1

We wish this book were out of date. We wish that the phenomenon of which it speaks—plant closings and their human consequences—had ceased to be. Instead, the book chronicles what was, at the time, the largest series of plant closings by a single employer—General Motors' 1987 plant closings. These closings promised job losses of 29,000, largely concentrated in the Rust Belt of Michigan and its environs.

This book tells a story of losses. When workers' jobs are lost, or even threatened, they pay an economic and emotional price. Their financial security is shaken. Their home life may be racked by strife between parent and child and between partner and partner. And their peace of mind—their sense of balance between the stresses of life and their ability to cope with those stresses—is disturbed.

This book also tells a story of strengths. We argue that it is part of the human condition to be susceptible to distress—to depression and anxiety, despair and fear—when objective circumstances are bad enough. We will seek both the causes and the cures of these workers' woes in the economic and social cards life deals them.

One message which emerges is that stress in life is unevenly distributed. Certain workers are better prepared to cope with the financial troubles that accompany a plant closing than others. Some have more money to start with, like high income workers. Some have more of a chance to regain jobs, or feel they do, like better educated or high seniority workers. Certain workers are likely to be facing more troubles in life anyway—whether or not a plant closes. And if these workers just happen to find themselves more often in a closing plant, life has just hit them with a double whammy. As later chapters will outline, some workers had it relatively easy or brutally rough simply because of who they were, or who they were *in combination with* where they were (in a closing plant, and then unemployed).

One of the things that gives people reason to believe is what they can see in themselves: what resources they have, what drawbacks they will acknowledge, what past they can draw on for comfort and what future they can envision for hope. In later chapters we also look into workers' thoughts and feelings about themselves and their lives. Here we find certain psychological strengths, such as the ability to cope with the situation in a way that offers hope and some semblance of a sense of control over fate. Within limits, what people believe to be true shapes what is true.

Other reasons to believe come from the world around us, from our intimate and not so intimate social ties. People don't solve the great crises of life alone, no matter what their collection of badges of status and worth. Blue–collar workers are no exception. Workers have several traditional means of coping with tragedy. One is religion, a cry for help directed upward. Another is loved ones and friends, the sort of help that can be found around one's own back yard. Yet another is a labor organization. Each of these means is in some sense collective, whether it refers to the bonds of a religious community, the arms of those who care about us most, or the brotherhood of those who share our way of making a living in this world. Other ways of getting help such as seeing a mental health professional, in contrast, focus on the individual who is in trouble. But when plants close down, the trouble that ensues is collective trouble.

When a crisis strikes we need all the help we can get. Our concluding arguments will focus on the necessity of combating the impact of plant closings through multiple factors, but especially the collective forces our workers drew upon for strength. When woes are spread across a plant, a state, or a nation, many forces come together to explain the resilience of those workers who survive the crisis and the despair of the rest. What gives hope is an amalgam, a combination, of reasons to believe in the self and the future. Much of the help is collective. It is drawn from other people and groups. Help comes to workers from those they love, from a God they worship actively, and from the union to which they belong. But for some, the sense of self, the experience of coping with negative events over a lifetime, and a resilience contributes greatly to the way in which they deal with the stress of the plant closing. The events of which we speak and study here occur at multiple levels—the micro– and macro levels. One of the features of this study is a bridging of the gap between these two levels to make sense of what happened to these workers and why it happened.

MICRO VERSUS MACRO APPROACHES

The meaning of the findings of social science can be sought along two dimensions: the macro versus the micro and the general versus the particular. The macro–micro distinction reflects the level of analysis taken by the author. An event like the 1987 General Motors plant closings takes place at multiple levels and has multiple meanings when looked at through the lens of the various social sciences. To economists, political scientists, and many sociologists, the 1987 General Motors plant closings are part of the story of the restructuring of the American economy in the latter decades of the twentieth century. This process, which at first seemed largely confined to blue–collar workers and their industries, has increasingly taken on a more general character and has become a threat to the middle class, as well as the working class (Bluestone & Harrison, 1982; Herz, 1991; Lobo & Watkins, 1995). It is commonplace now to speak of past, present, and potential future "downsizing" on the part of American industry and the corporate world.

This way of looking at the event is extremely important in its own right. Our focus, however, lies at the level of the individual worker who, like the workers quoted at the start of this chapter, finds that the world has gone topsy–turvy and cannot be made right. This book is intended to be a microlevel counterpart to those studies that look at industrial transformation. We ask what happens to individuals:

whether they get reemployed, how, and when;

how they feel and think—whether, for example, they suffer from depression or anxiety;

and what happens to their family life.

Ours is a study of stress which tries to situate the stressful experience within the life course and the social world of those affected. This kind of investigation stands at the crossroads of psychology and sociology.

The second dimension on which works can be arrayed, the general versus the particular, refers to the degree to which the macro– or microlevel topic is being investigated in its unique particulars or for its general characteristics. For example, our microlevel study concerns stress, but inevitably it is also a study of stress in particular circumstances: a particular time and place, among people of a certain occupation, and certain other social characteristics. Research always has a greater or lesser degree of generalizability; it correspondingly reveals, depending on the fineness of the knife with which the investigator has cut, a greater or lesser degree of specificity of message.

The interplay between general and particular is central to our attempt to fuse stress models with the burgeoning literature on the life course. Stress is a familiar term in several of the social and medical sciences, as will be discussed later in this chapter. The "life course" is a newer and less familiar one. The outlines of the perspective are presented more fully from a number of recent works, notably those of Glen Elder (Elder, 1985, 1994; Elder & O'Rand, 1995). To situate our study of the stress of unemployment in the life course literature is to adopt certain ways of thinking about history and social structure. First and foremost, such a perspective emphasizes ways in which the smooth flow of individual lives can be interrupted, bent, and sometimes broken by the history in which they are embedded. Related to this, it becomes important to ask how lives which are intertwined are mutually affected: How does the job loss of husband affect wife, or the job loss of parent affect child? And finally, the "focal victim" (here, the job loser) has personal and social characteristics that make the meeting with history a more or less difficult proposition. For example, studies of the life course have shown that when people undergo a predictable life transition at an unexpected time (as when older men were drafted to serve in World War II), stress is greater (Elder, 1986; 1987; Hogan, 1981). And sometimes such characteristics as age or gender or social class change the meaning of a crisis. Elder's classic study *Children of the Great Depression* (1974), for example, found that adjustment to hard times in the Great Depression was easier for older children and for boys, who were able to work outside the home and contribute to family income.

What the life course literature helps to do is to emphasize the particularity of any given crisis and any given group visited by it. History is always particular and multiply so. Whereas we might wish to make pronouncements and draw conclusions about the "nature of stress," what we are faced with are concrete, specific realities. Concreteness can characterize both the macro– and the micro level. The 1987 General Motors plant closings were, at the macro level, a particular example of the process of downsizing, a particular instance of the labor relations of one company and its work force. At the microlevel, these closings provided evidence about the nature of stress, indeed, and about the more specific nature of stress as it is experienced among the unemployed. But most concretely, the stresses were those of particular workers with histories, resources, weaknesses, and strengths, who had come into the auto factories at a particular point in history and exited at the special juncture of the late 1980s. At its core, the life course perspective is about the ways in which history and biography interact.

Theoretically and methodologically, this is a microlevel study whose main thrust is toward identifying general trends and effects. Our methodology, survey research, is well suited to exploring general microlevel trends (see Chapter Two). We shall use insights from the stress and life course literatures to make it possible to explore particularities as well. The most consistent theme will be the interaction between the stressor and the people who experience it. This is couched in terms of the presence or absence of various resources which enable the workers to be more or less resistant to the stress and strain of unemployment and its threat. Unemployment constitutes "hard times"; shortages of social, economic, and personal resources make for "vulnerable people." Unemployment, like other stressors, does not affect its victims equally; it is when hard times meet vulnerable people that the toll occurs.

We will return to the life course perspective and its overlap with the literature on stress after considering more fully what it means to say that the closing of an auto plant or the loss of a job is stressful, and why we should care that it is so.

STRESS AND COPING MODELS

The general conception of stress used in this and other research on stressful events comes from the seminal work of Hans Selye (1956, 1976). In early work, Selye laid out what he termed the General Adaptation Syndrome to describe the stages of stress. These stages are (1) *alarm*, in which the threat/harm is perceived and the animal mobilizes; (2) *resistance*, in which the animal defends against a continued threat; and (3) *exhaustion*, in which the body fails. Although he initially met with resistance and even derision for his work, Selye's own output of hundreds of books and thousands of articles plus the growing body of work done worldwide have made the notion of stress a medical commonplace and also a coffee–table companion for many of us moderns.

The Stress Process

Increasingly the stress process as a whole is viewed as an interaction between person and environment, a matter of balance between the demands imposed by the environment and the resources the person has or can call upon for meeting those demands (e.g., Hobfoll, 1988, 1989; Kessler, Price, & Wortman, 1985). The literature can be divided into approaches that emphasize the objective qualities of the environment that cause stress versus approaches that emphasize the perceptions and vulnerabilities of the individual subjected to the stressor. Interestingly enough, recent research on both sides of that divide appears to be reaching a consensus in which the generally held view is that objective circumstances differ reliably in their stressfulness and that individual differences in perception are vitally important.

Perhaps the best illustration of this rapproachment is the area of life events research. In the early days in which Holmes and Rahe (1967) had just developed their scale of putatively stressful life events, there was an enormous rush of empirical research; its result, all too often, was to demonstrate a modest relationship between the occurrence of various events and such negative outcomes as depression. Researchers quickly realized that they could get a more differentiated picture by finding out more from the individual about the event, and just as quickly, they saw that this put them into a potentially unenviable vicious circle. Those people who saw events as more stressful indeed tended to be more depressed, and so forth, but the depression could obviously be the cause of this relationship as easily as it was the effect. (For discussions see Brown & Harris, 1978; Dohrenwend & Dohrenwend, 1981; Thoits, 1983.) One result is that researchers such as Brown and Harris have been working intensively on interviews that can capture specific aspects of events but are not contaminated by depression.

A second strand of objective determinants considered in the stress process is the resources the person possesses: economic, social, psychological, physical, or whatever. Hobfoll (1988; 1989) is one psychological theorist who has emphasized resources. By taking into account demographic characteristics, many sociologists are implicitly or explicitly "resource" theorists (e.g., Kessler et al., 1985; Pearlin, 1989). Demographic and other resources play a couple of major roles. Either they serve to make the person more or less likely to be stressed in the first place ("exposure"), or they serve to make the person more or less susceptible to the stressor once it is experienced ("vulnerability" or "reactivity").

The most firmly subjectivist approach to stress is that of Richard Lazarus, writing on his own or with co–authors, most notably Susan Folkman (Lazarus & Folkman, 1984). Lazarus has consistently emphasized that the crucial feature to understanding stress response is individual differences and that these individual differences can be studied in terms of what he calls appraisal and coping.

Our own stress model builds on the work of Leonard Pearlin, a sociologist; we see his model as a hybrid between the objectivist and subjectivist camps. He emphasizes the importance of background factors, but often sees them as governing perceptions and reactions (i.e., such aspects as appraisal and coping). The next series of figures serve to illustrate how a complex, socio–psychological model can be built up from the simple relationship between stressor and reaction to it.

Figure 1.1 shows the simplest version of the stress process. It is a kind of "black box" model as in the early days of learning theory, in that it makes no assumptions or predictions about what goes on in the head of the person under stress. It is basically tautological: A stressor appears, a reaction occurs, and the observer concludes that an instance of "stress" has occurred. We see no way, for example, to explore how some people may respond much more extremely to the stressor than others or how some stressors are generally more difficult to cope with, and so forth. We simply have the basic framework: stressor in, stress process (inferred), reactions out.

Figure 1.2 begins our expansion of this black box, first in a backward direction. It attempts to indicate some of the reasons why Person A and Person B can react so differently to the "same" event. The basic categories of reasons are twofold, as we have noted: differential *exposure* and *reactivity* or vulnerability. We shall reserve discussion of particular examples of vulnerability that interest us here for later (in a discussion of moderator variables; Fig. 1.4), because sources of vulnerability fit statistically and logically into the category of moderator effects.

Figure 1.3 begins to address what happens "within the box" itself: what are the differences in the meaning of the stimulus or its processing that can help to account for differential response and recovery. This figure summarizes the meaning of the particular stressor under study here: unemployment.

We argue that loss (or anticipated loss) of work has stressful effects through two major pathways:

1. Objectively, job loss brings on financial hardship to individuals and families. (Pearlin, Lieberman, Menaghan, & Mullan's, 1981 model of the process also included income loss at this stage, so their path went job loss—> income loss ——> financial hardship. We have chosen a more simplified presentation given the number of variables we wish to include at the various stages.)

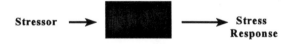

Figure 1.1. Stressor and stress response as a "black box".

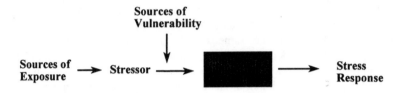

Figure 1.2. Expanding the black box backward: predictors of stress exposure and vulnerability.

    2. Subjectively, job loss itself and financial hardships that ensue can each erode the worker's sense of self–worth and self–control.

    In Pearlin et al.'s (1981) models these two constructs were represented by scales of self–esteem and mastery.   These specific constructs and their measurement will be discussed further below and will be the subject of a chapter in their own right. For present purposes, what is important is the idea that job loss has negative effects on people for both financial and psychological reasons.
    Other stressors may activate a different complex of thoughts and feelings; for example, a nonfinancial stressor may not be mediated by thoughts about financial hardship at all.   In general, however, we shall argue that self–worth and self–efficacy are among the "master paths" of meaning through which a variety of stressors wreak their havoc.

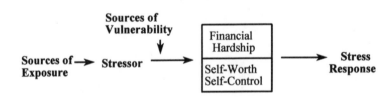

Figure 1.3. Inside the black box I: mediators of stress response in the case of unemployment.

For different stressors, different mediators might be appropriate, reflecting the different meanings of these stressful events or circumstances. Figure 1.4 depicts a more complex relationship inside the "box." The variables added to the model here are shown above and below the causal line between stressor and response, and the arrows from them come down to touch the cause–effect line itself to illustrate that they are moderators of the stress response. A moderator variable changes the nature of the relationship between the variable that precedes and the variable that follows it; the moderator itself need not have any particular relationship to the effect (here, the stress response).

Figure 1.4 depicts three important types of moderator variables. First, we have already mentioned that certain demographic characteristics may be associated with differential reactivity or vulnerability to certain stressors, that is, certain demographics may moderate the impact of unemployment or other stressful circumstances. The two upon which we shall concentrate are *gender* and *race*; these issues are briefly summarized in the chapter outline that follows, and the results of our analyses about gender and race appear in Chapter Five.

The second broad category of moderator is coping styles or decisions. Most of the literature on coping has focused on how people approach a stressor. The most common distinction, for example, is that between *problem*–focused coping and *emotion*–focused coping (Lazarus & Folkman, 1984); people can either attempt to change the situation or attempt to change their emotional reaction to it. Our primary focus will instead be the decisions people make about whether they are looking for work or not and the fit between decision and outcome. Our basic argument will be that outcomes that allow the person to retain a sense of control tend to be beneficial, whether or not these outcomes are conventionally those thought of as problem–solving.

The third type of moderator is social support, reviewed in Chapter Nine. For example, previous literature on unemployment and on work–related stress has generally (although not always) found that workers who have some source of social support, often a spouse, are less badly impacted by the financially related stress associated with work and work loss. Our discussion of social support will also be expanded to take into account the effects of getting professional help, as well as the effects of collective supports such as union and church. In each case, the key question about this factor as a moderator is whether the person who has the support (or a greater amount of it) is more resistant to the stressor and/or more rapidly recovers from it.

There is one final direction in which to expand the black box of stress: forward to consider its multiple consequences and their sequelae. A whole family of distressful consequences can follow from a stressor like unemployment; like the rest of the book, this chapter concentrates on mental health consequences. Family consequences are also a common focus of unemployment research, in that the family itself can be damaged or destroyed (separation, divorce), the other individuals in it (spouse, children) can suffer from stress and develop stress–related disease outcomes, and the nature of interaction among family members can deteriorate. The book's secondary focus is the stability of family life; thirdly, we will briefly address such topics as workers' health, drinking and drug use, and family members' physical health. Figure 1.5 highlights the primary consequences we study.

Finally, stressful situations do not simply end as if they were scenes from a play, after which "real life" can simply resume; instead, the life of a worker who goes through a crisis like the plant closings we studied may be changed forever. The trajectory of life is altered because future job searches carry with them the baggage of and fallout from the job loss. Therefore, the ultimate consequence of a major stressful experience such as unemployment therefore is to be found in the reverberating themes and the interacting threads of subsequent lives.

Figure 1.6 provides an illustrative example. It treats depression and family stress as initial consequences of unemployment and then traces a probable sequence for the way these may feed into (and impede) subsequent reemployment. Its message is straightforward. The person who becomes unemployed is more likely to experience distress of various kinds, including anxiety, depression, and hostility. For reasons we spell out in later chapters, we view depression and anxiety as the central forms of distress that carry forth into later events and circumstances, but theoretically any kind of distress will do. Simply put, to have become unemployed and hence distressed—depressed, anxious, whatever—is to be less likely to gain reemployment or more likely to lose a subsequent job. Unemployment deals a

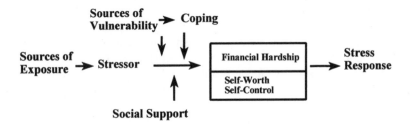

Figure 1.4. Inside the black box II: moderators of stress response.

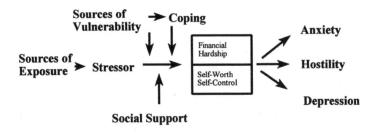

Figure 1.5. Expanding the black box forward: consequences of stress.

double whammy because its consequence, distress, has further
consequences—reduced employability—which make it harder to get back to square
unemployment leads to family stress and disruption, this too can have
consequences
for future employment, if only because it too feeds the spiral of distress. Even the
most "event–like" of life disruptions are in fact processes which have antecedents,

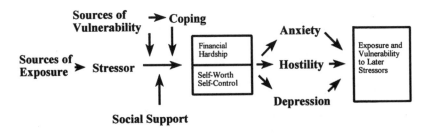

Figure 1.6. Linkages among the black boxes: stress consequences become part
of subsequent stress processes.

concomitants, and sequelae; even though unemployment occurs on a specific day at a specific time, for its duration, it is a state as well as an event.

Events versus Processes

Many stressors like unemployment can be thought of in terms of both discrete events and the continuous processes those events unleash. In fact, the recent literature has often distinguished between discrete, acutely stressful events and continuous, chronically stressful processes. Recently Pearlin (1989) and others have become more interested in the impact of chronic stressors. Such activities as caregiving for someone with Alzheimer's or AIDS prove to be extraordinarily stressful. One reason is the fact that as they unfold, the original stressors generate subsequent stressors. Pearlin (1989) captured this distinction in the terms *primary* versus *secondary* stressor. A secondary stressor may be as big as the initial one, or bigger; its "secondary" status is indicative of its position in the causal sequence, not of its potency. For caregivers, strains at work tend to follow from the time and energy they spend in caregiving. The secondary and primary strains, together, contribute to the overall stress response.

Although the primary–secondary stressor distinction is important in the stress literature, the time line of our unemployment cases is short enough that we adopt the language of the more abbreviated original "stress process" model depicted in Figure 1.5 (Pearlin et al., 1981; discussed below). In that model, stressors produce effects that mediate between the stressor and the outcomes. Mediators occupy the same logical position in the original stress model that secondary stressors do in the recent modifications.

Our conclusion (Chapter Ten) provides an overview of our results and raises some implications of our work for the study of the stress process. For present purposes, the major message of our research is twofold:

1. *Life's events, crises, and phases are both sequenced and interconnected,*
2. *Human fates in a family or community are interdependent, intertwined by both the causes that impinge upon them and the effects they feel.*

In this case, the event—the stressor— is actual or anticipated unemployment. Unemployment as a life event (or process) has long been known to have important consequences for individuals and their families. It is important to take into account what is already known about what unemployment does to people and their loved ones before we embark on what could be seen as yet another study of a well–known problem. The next section reviews unemployment research in greater detail, closing with a summary of ways in which the current study is distinctive. The chapter concludes with a summary of the book's goals and the organization of the later chapters.

UNEMPLOYMENT AS A STRESSOR

Since the 1930s, social scientists have been demonstrating that unemployment is a stressor for workers and their families. Unemployment is considered a highly stressful, negative life event (Dohrenwend, Krasnoff, Askenasy, & Dohrenwend, 1978), with good reason: Studies of both general unemployment and plant closings show that unemployment is associated with a significant increase in symptoms such as perceived physical illness, hostility, paranoia, drinking problems, family conflict, and demoralization, as well as depression, anxiety, and somatic symptoms (Buss & Redburn, 1983; Dooley & Catalano, 1988; Feather, 1990; Jahoda, 1982; Kelvin & Jarrett, 1985; Kessler, House, & Turner, 1987; Kessler, Turner, & House, 1987, 1988; Pearlin et al., 1981; Perrucci, Perrucci, Targ, & Targ, 1988; Warr, 1987). The key question that researchers must address is whether the unemployment really *caused* the negative outcome. This turns out to be a complex and not easily answered question.

Marienthal, an early landmark, was an in–depth study of a town in Austria that experienced very high unemployment during the Depression (Jahoda, Lazarsfeld, & Zeisel, 1933). The authors conceptualized unemployment as following a sequence analogous to the stages of grieving over a loved one. They set a standard for later research in the meticulous attention they paid to various kinds of data, both qualitative and quantitative, and in their treatment of unemployment as a family rather than an individual problem. They lacked, however, many of the standard aids to inference that they would have had in doing a classic laboratory experiment; they were doing work that was more like an epidemiological investigation of an epidemic, and the epidemic in question affected a large percentage of the population. Their task was more one of documenting a phenomenon than of establishing its origins. Another way to describe the situation is that they had one research "subject"—the town of Marienthal.

Like *Marienthal*, most studies of unemployment have had to use case study methods or cross–sectional surveys. Case studies are particularly logical designs when entire geographical regions are affected, as in a plant closing or other mass layoff. The social scientist interviews workers whose plant is about to shut down or has already done so. Interviews are usually repeated, often include family members other than the workers themselves, and can include information about the larger community or town and effects of the plant closing on the entire scene. Buss and Redburn's (1983) work in Youngstown, Ohio; Kathryn Dudley's (1994) work, and Ruth Milkman's (1997) exploration of the plant closing in Linden, New Jersey; Greg Pappas's (1989) research in Barberton, Ohio; and the Perrucci et al. (1988) study of a shutdown in Monticello, Indiana, by RCA are classic examples of the case study method that span sociological and anthropological approaches.

In the cross–sectional survey, employed and unemployed workers are compared at a particular point in time. An obvious weakness of this method, of course, is that we do not know certainly whether the unemployment causes the observed differences, is the effect of the differences, or some mixture of the two. In recent decades, survey studies of unemployment have usually attempted to gather data at more than one point (although usually broad–based surveys are unable to catch people both before and during a spell of unemployment because of the statistical rarity of unemployment); for examples, see Pearlin et al. (1981) and the research program by Kessler and his colleagues (Kessler et al., 1987a, 1987b, 1988).

It is partly the "purity" of the event in causal terms that attracts social scientists to plant closings and other incidents of mass worker displacement. Such events are often known about enough in advance that some measurement can be taken before the unemployment begins—although usually not before the knowledge of impending unemployment has been communicated to the worker. No one can accomplish the purity of a laboratory experiment in the case of unemployment because people cannot be randomly assigned to gain or lose jobs, but a mass job loss can reasonably be considered to be something beyond the worker's control. We get to observe the effects of unemployment on various worker characteristics with a certain amount of confidence that the worker characteristic has not itself brought on the unemployment. (For further discussion of methodological issues and of experimental design, see Chapter Two; for unemployment as a cause of mental distress, see Chapter Four and Hamilton et al., 1993.)

The optimal kind of study for teasing out the ways in which unemployment causes difficulties is the quasi–experiment, in which groups of workers are compared: one group that is (or is about to become) unemployed, and a second group that is not. This kind of design is remarkably rare. The landmark study of this type is Cobb & Kasl's (1977) *Termination*, a study of plant closings, which Chapter Two will review. Our research also follows a quasi–experimental logic in comparing groups that are and are not subject to plant shutdowns and in interviewing them both before and (twice) after the plants have closed.

As a stressor, unemployment has several features that draw social scientists to it for scientific as well as policy reasons. Scientifically, it is a known stressor, a serious one, and a stressor that under certain circumstances—such as a quasi–experiment—can be fairly cleanly isolated and studied for its effects. Ethically and politically, it has such widespread and negative effects on entire populations that it is a question of public policy, not just of science, to ask how it works and wreaks its damage.

Consequences of the Stress Process

Stress has been implicated as a cause of or contributor to a dizzying array of physical, mental, and interpersonal bad outcomes (e.g., Cassel, 1976; Selye, 1956). We had certain specific areas in which it was possible to gather data on auto workers affected by plant closings. It is these areas that are featured in this book.

For two reasons, our interest centers on mental health and particularly on the arena of mood and anxiety disorders. These appear to be the "common cold" of reactions to stress—a very common type of outcome; and they manifest themselves quickly, soon enough to be picked up in a research project of only a couple of years' duration. It is possible that the workers whom we studied will eventually show a higher incidence of cardiac problems, ulcers, or cancer, but we are not likely to be able to document it in the short time frame (a bit more than two years) in which we worked.

We had a secondary interest in family stress, including reactions of both spouse and children to the unemployment experience. This arena is secondary for practical rather than intellectual reasons. We interviewed only workers, not workers and their families. Thus, if we heard about a distressed spouse or child, it was via the worker; the evidence is second–hand.

Four basic types of mental distress are tapped: depression, anxiety, hostility, and somatic complaints. As later discussions will spell out, somatic complaints are a kind of "control group" in this case, complaints that are not strongly related to the stressor in question (unemployment). Hostility also plays a secondary role in our research; as Chapter Seven will show, it is related more strongly to a past stressor (military combat) than it is to the one we were studying (unemployment). The key outcomes, those that often earn such terms as the "common cold" of mental disorders, are anxiety and depression.

Empirically, anxiety and depression are closely linked. Many studies that use checklists or questionnaire measures find that the two are strongly related (correlations on the order of .75 or .8 are not uncommon). Theoretically, in most current approaches to these two forms of distress, there is a common thread: anxiety is the leading edge, in that it represents a reaction to a threat of loss (or of that loss's aftereffects); depression is the lagging indicator, in that depression conceptually represents reaction to the loss itself. The anxious person feels *helpless*; the depressed person, *hopeless* (Garber, Miller, & Abramson, 1980). In the chapters that follow, we explore the basic logic of anxiety, depression, hostility, and "anxious depression" by relating them to a limited set of concepts:

loss (and its threat)
worth
control
blame

We draw upon several different theories in coming to this set of concepts. Loss and threat are notions so general that they pervade the literature. From the sociological literature, specifically the Pearlin et al. (1981) model to be presented later, we take the notion that a person's self–esteem (worth; Rosenberg, 1965) and sense of mastery (control) are crucial intervening factors that turn a negative event into a negative mental health state. The notion that blame is central takes different forms for different mood states. Specifically, hostility is viewed as blame directed outward, whereas depression has been viewed as blame directed inward. Aaron Beck's (1967, 1976, 1987) cognitive therapy for depression also emphasizes self–blame as a key component of depression (in addition to hopelessness and worthlessness).

As we conceptualize it, a loss/threat event sets in motion a series of reactions, some truncated or elongated version of Selye's General Adaptation Syndrome, coupled with emotional reactions. Anxiety is the emotion of the hunter waiting for the boar to erupt from the tall grass. Its terribly maladaptive quality in our modern world is that some boars wait for years. We view the main path to pain in the case of anxiety as flowing through control. The person who is anxious is afraid of being unable to cope with a hidden, imagined, or fully–in–view wild boar. We agree with Bandura (1977) that anxiety has effects on the sense of control (what Bandura terms self–efficacy) and conversely that self–efficacy protects against anxiety.

In contrast, a key element in hostility is the fact that the person blames other(s) for the loss or threat of loss. Anger is directed externally.

Depression, finally, involves the person's senses of worth, control, and self–blame. A reduced sense of self–worth is almost certainly present (Beck, 1967); helplessness or diminished sense of control is commonly felt (see Seligman, 1975; Abrahamson, Seligman, & Teasdale, 1978); and in the long run depression is likely to incorporate elevated self–blame.

It is easy to see how anxiety and depression can be intertwined, given these contributing forces. Many times anxiety, roused by a threat, is maintained during a loss; and the loss of control that engenders and is engendered by anxiety feeds the depression that ensues. The person ends up an "anxious depressive." It will be our contention that this is the basic sequence in the stressful circumstances surrounding unemployment, and this is the reason why studies in this field so routinely find anxiety and depression increasing in tandem.

The stress model we adopt primarily follows the lines of Figure 1.5 with some attention to the longer term outgrowths of unemployment in Figure 1.6. It attempts to explore how certain facts of life such as financial hardship and the attendant feelings, reduced self–worth, loss of control, or increased self–blame, can mediate and moderate the response to job loss or its threat *among a certain group of workers with their personal mixes of resources and vulnerabilities to hard times.*

OVERVIEW OF THE BOOK

The ensuing chapters are arranged in a circle. After an introduction to the methodology of the study in Chapter Two, we turn first to the basic outcomes of the unemployment we studied, characterized in terms of consequences for jobs and reemployment (Chapter Three), for mental health, and for family life and its stresses (Chapter Four).

Given these end points, we loop back to work our way through the stress process as it has been outlined in Chapter One. We first consider how worker's characteristics influence their experience of unemployment in Chapter Five. Our central foci are race and gender. Chapter Six begins our discussion of mediators and moderators. Given that a stressor—unemployment—has been identified and its key consequences outlined, the first question is what mediating factors we can identify. In other words, how does unemployment do the damage it does? The key mediators, according to the original Pearlin et al. (1981) model, can be expected to be financial hardship on the one hand and aspects of self–concept, particularly self–esteem and mastery or self–efficacy, on the other. Chapter Six addresses these financial and self–related impacts of unemployment. We concentrate on the mediation of mental health outcomes, both here and elsewhere in discussing the stress process.

Chapter Seven addresses previous or concurrent negative life events, particularly military service and combat experience. Here we consider the issue of carryover stress and its relationship to unemployment. We seek to extend the conceptualization of the stress process.

The most commonly studied moderators of the stress process are factors that can be introduced or drawn upon to ameliorate or buffer the impact of stress. Chapters Eight and Nine turn to two key categories of potential buffers: cognitive strategies for dealing with the stressor (Chapter Eight) and social support, or helpseeking, from others (Chapter Nine).

The conclusion, Chapter Ten, draws together the strands of the model, as developed thus far, to yield an overall statement. Its key message is that the impact of even a powerful stressor like unemployment is distinctly *contextual*, linked to who the person was before the stressor hit and what resources the person has to draw upon to recover from that stressor. It is also *historical*, in that the meaning of the event depends on its place in history. In this case, for example, the unemployment was not the routine humdrum sort of unemployment that American autoworkers have long become used to as model years change and tail fins are replaced. It was seen by many workers as a sea change in worker–management relationships, a fundamental alteration in the agreement under which they worked the line for pay. The bottom line is that the downsizing of the factory offers a model of the way stress invades the lives of individuals in large and subtle ways, depending upon who the person is. Under some circumstances, for some workers, job loss during downsizing makes barely a dent; for other workers, or under different circumstances, job loss savages the worker's planned life trajectory, the worker's peace of mind and spirit, and the harmony of the worker's home.

Now tragedy is a textured thing. Stressors in the current era are every bit as serious as the wild boar that once hid in the brush. But they are now fundamentally social: dependent for their meaning and impact on human interpretations of their existence and seriousness. It is the job of social scientists to find the clues about ways to combat the new, uniquely human crises that we must meet now.

2

The Study: Sites, Sample, Method, and Measures

On November 6, 1986, General Motors announced that it would be closing nine plants and parts of two others by 1990, most by the end of 1987. This announcement represented a major blow to the state of Michigan, which had the highest concentration of plants, and to the members of the International Union, United Automobile, Aerospace, and Agricultural Implement Workers of America (UAW), who would take the brunt of the job losses. Early in 1987, the Michigan Health and Social Security Research Institute, founded and operated by the UAW, began a study of individuals and families who would be affected by 1987 GM shutdowns.

This chapter describes the *where* of the plant closing study: the sites where GM plants were scheduled to close, as well as a detailed picture of *who* was studied ("the sample") and *how* we studied them ("method and measures").

THE SITES

The Closing Plants

Four closing plants in Michigan were geographically convenient for us to study: one GM plant in Flint (the Buick–Oldsmobile–Cadillac Assembly plant) and three in Detroit (Clark Street, Fleetwood, and Fort Street).

Fleetwood and Clark Street. Within the city limits of Detroit, on Clark and Fort Streets, stood the Fleetwood complex. The original facility was built in 1916 by the federal government. Its purpose had been the construction of aircraft for the

World War I mobilization effort. By the end of 1918, more than two thousand aircraft had come across its assembly line. In fact, this facility pioneered the development of assembly line practices for the mass production of transportation equipment in the United States. After the war, the facility was reconstructed to suit the needs of automobile manufacturing. A six–story addition was added in 1922, and in 1926 it became part of General Motors when the corporation purchased Fisher Body. In the Fleetwood/Clark Street complex's two million square feet, spread out over 45 acres, General Motors then manufactured Cadillac bodies for its top of the line vehicles.

The complex included the Cadillac assembly plant, a bumper plating operation, and extensive administrative offices.   It was the home of the classic rear–wheel–drive Cadillac brougham. Bodies were built at the Fleetwood end of the complex and then transported to Clark Street for mounting and assembly of the finished product. The three–mile hiatus between the body and finished product assembly locations made the operation costly and inefficient. So, after building more than seven million vehicles since the 1920s, GM began to shift work to a newer facility in Arlington, Texas, in 1986. Final closing of Fleetwood and Clark Street occurred in December 1987.

Fort Street. The Fort Street Plant, or Fisher Guide as it was more commonly called, was a component parts manufacturing facility. Rather than being a body or chassis construction site, this was a feeder plant. Smaller component parts for doors, interiors, roofs, and dozens of other hardware products in more than 10,000 configurations were manufactured here and supplied the assembly lines at other General Motors facilities.

Fort Street had kept pace with the times technologically. As recently as 1984, it had served as the host consolidation site after the closing of six other Fisher Body hardware plant operations. However, the hourly work force at this plant dwindled through the years, down from a high of over 2,000 permanent employees to about 1,400 workers by late 1987. All production at the plant ceased at the end of the workday on Friday, June 16, 1989.

Flint's B–O–C Assembly (originally Fisher Body No. 1). This plant went by various names over the years, but to the workers it came to be referred to, most of the time, as "Fisher One." Standing on Saginaw Street on the outskirts of Flint, Michigan, the plant was expanded and transformed during the 1930s into the largest facility in the world for building car bodies. It originally produced bodies for Buick Motor Company, later becoming a part of General Motors.

As early as the 1930s, the plant employed several thousand workers. More than 10 million auto bodies were produced at Fisher Body No. 1 between World War II and the mid–1980s. But because the facility was old and new technologies had not been integrated into its physical plant, the number of employees declined dramatically by the late 1970s.

THE HISTORICAL CONTEXT

The workers who punched in at Clark Street, Fleetwood, and Fisher One on December 10, 1987, the last hours of their operation, labored under a burden of history. This was true at Clark Street and Fleetwood, which had participated in the 1936–1937 sit–down strike in which the UAW won recognition from GM, and it was especially true at Fisher One, which had been the heart of the strike. Workers at Fisher One saw their plant as special, and they saw its closure as having a particularly bitter meaning. Many wore T–shirts to commemorate their loss, carrying messages like: "1937 SIT–DOWN, 1987 SHUT–DOWN" and "FISHER 1—GONE BUT NOT FORGOTTEN."

Rightly or wrongly, workers did take the loss of their plant as having historical significance. Their loss was not an individual, personal one—or not only that. It was a collective loss to members of a union. The rest of this book tells the story of what happened to these workers when the plants closed down.

The next part of this chapter addresses the question of how to measure best the effects of the plant closing. An important part of the answer is that one must also look at workers in other plants which did *not* close. Therefore we also studied 12 nonclosing plants, as discussed further here.   Throughout the book, these comparison plants will remain unnamed, anonymous counterparts to Clark Street, Fleetwood, Fort Street, and Fisher One.

STUDYING THE EFFECTS OF PLANT CLOSINGS

The closing of a plant has effects on individuals, their families, their communities, and the economies that once depended on the output of those plants. We focus at the close–in, "hands–on" level of effects on individual workers and their family ties. There are three types of effects that we focus on in this book:

1. Financial consequences to workers and their families are almost inevitable. Plant closings hurt — not only workers who lose jobs, but also workers who keep their jobs. The latter may have jobs, but find that their sense of security is lost and their sense of financial well–being is cast in doubt. Chapter Three focuses on the impact of the GM plant closings on employment and Chapter Six addresses the implications of job loss: the variety of financial hardships to which workers might fall victim.

2. Mental health can be seriously affected by a plant closing. For example, research has shown that the mental health impact of unemployment includes increases in depression and anxiety. Losing a job does not usually make a person paranoid or catatonic, but it often leads to the panic of anxiety and the despair of depression. Because mental health effects can appear immediately,

even before plants actually close, we expected to find the most immediate and evident impact of the GM plant closings in this arena. After its introduction in Chapter Four, mental health is the core issue in most of the remaining chapters; it lies at the center of the stress model we have outlined.

3. Family consequences are probable but not certain under the circumstances of plant closing. These may include effects as mild as an increase in nitpicking or strained relationships within the family. Serious effects may include such outcomes as physical abuse or divorce. Chapter Four also traces the impact of the plant closings on workers' relationships within the family and on the health of family members. In the long run, we argue that there is a reciprocal relationship between the feelings of workers and those of their families: distressed workers make for strained family ties, and family strain generates distress.

Designing the Research Project

The main objective of the study was to estimate changes in individuals' and families' lives that could be clearly attributed to plant closings. We used a prospective quasi–experimental design to examine the impact of plant closings on workers and their families (Cook & Campbell, 1979). Our study compared workers from four closing plants with workers from 12 non-closing plants in the greater Detroit and Flint areas. The first phase, the gathering of baseline or "before" data, consisted of face-to-face interviews with 1,597 workers that took place approximately three months before the plant closings. The second wave of large–scale interviewing occurred in 1988, involving 1,288 workers, and the third in 1989, involving 1,136 workers. Finally, a small group of 30 workers who were identified as highly depressed or nondepressed on the basis of the three surveys were interviewed again during the summer of 1991 in an intensive, clinical–style, open–ended format. The latter interviews are the source of the quotes we use throughout the book.

In our study, we expected that workers in plants that were not closing might initially be affected—for example, might be more anxious than usual. Therefore, it must be remembered that the results we report are differences between a probably less than relaxed "control" group, who may fear future plant closings, and a group currently experiencing plant closure. Chapter Four documents the fact that "control group" workers whose plants did not close experienced distress at the start of our study.

Throughout the book, we refer to workers from nonclosing plants as a *comparison* group rather than a control group, to emphasize the fact that this is not a true experiment but a quasi–experiment in which everyone was susceptible to distress and fear of the future.

The Samples

Workers were randomly sampled from two groups: hourly workers at General Motors plants scheduled to close in December 1987 and hourly workers at General Motors plants not scheduled to close. Workers from Detroit's Clark Street, Fort Street, and Fleetwood plants and Flint's Fisher #1 Assembly Plant comprised the closing plant population. In actuality, the distinction between closing and nonclosing plants did not end up as clear–cut as we initially thought. The small Fort Street plant did not fully close until 1989. Also, one production line was closed at a "nonclosing" plant. However, we decided to compare these plants as originally designated. The population of non-closing plant workers consisted of workers from 12 GM plants not scheduled to close in the Metropolitan Detroit or Greater Flint areas that also met the following criteria:

greater than 100 employees;
demographically similar to closing plants;
not currently involved in a similar research project;
and not a warehouse or distribution center.

Thus the first stage of sampling, in which plants were chosen, was purposive rather than random. Although findings may be applicable to autoworkers in other locations, our study literally applies to GM workers in the Detroit and Flint areas.

How might this locale affect the results? The American auto industry developed in this region. Detroit, not Los Angeles, is the nation's Motown. These plant closings represented a threat not just to individual jobs but to a regional economy and a blue–collar style of life. In both closing and nonclosing plants, autoworkers had grown up in an environment in which autos provided well–paying, secure employment for the blue–collar worker.

In Detroit, Flint, and other industrial cities of the Midwest, the auto plants have been a family affair for more than 50 years. More than half of all the workers we studied had parents who were autoworkers. Furthermore, more than 30% had grandparents who were autoworkers. Approximately 10% had other household members who currently worked at automobile plants. Of those with household members (including spouses) who worked at auto plants, approximately one-third worked in the same plant. For workers with such family histories, employment in the automotive industry may be an important part of the worker's family history and identity, and plant closing may take a particularly heavy toll. Even workers whose plants do not close are aware that options for their children and grandchildren are disappearing.

Paradoxically, the importance of this industry to the workforce and the importance of these plants to the workers probably means that this book's assertions about the effect of plant closing are underestimates. This is true because we test for an effect of the closings by comparing workers from closing plants with others whose plants did not close. And these comparison group workers may themselves be affected—afraid, unhappy, or despairing.

Choosing the Samples: Wave 1. After selecting the plants to be included in the study, a sample of individual workers was drawn from General Motors' June 6, 1987 payroll. Only those recorded on the payroll as "actively employed" or "laid off" from closing plants, or "actively employed" from nonclosing plants were included in the sample frame. All workers from closing plants with definite plans to transfer to another plant were excluded from the study. Workers on military, personal, sick, or disability leave, as well as retirees were also excluded.

To secure interviews with approximately 1,600 workers, 6,400 names (3,200 from each group) were randomly drawn. We anticipated that as many as four names would be needed for every completed interview, because of incomplete information on the payroll listing, as well as various forms of nonresponse. This estimate proved accurate. No telephone numbers and addresses were available for 2,835 of those sampled, although every attempt was made to locate telephone numbers for each sampled name.

Comparison of Nonclosing and Closing Plant Workers. How did closing plant workers differ from workers in plants that were not scheduled to close? Because the research was a quasi–experiment rather than an experiment, any initial differences between workers in one group and workers in the other were important to know about.

In Wave 1, we examined a number of personal characteristics that could themselves produce financial hardship, family strife, and poor physical or mental health. Those characteristics that seemed most likely to have such an effect were age, gender, race, marital status, seniority at GM, annual wage, and skill level. For example, younger, lower seniority, and unskilled workers could be expected to have lower wages at the outset, and lower wages, in turn, would generate financial hardship.

Table 2.1 highlights the contrasts; it shows several important differences between workers from closing plants and workers from nonclosing plants.

Closing plant workers, who were at a much higher risk of losing their jobs, were disproportionately female, nonwhite, unmarried, and young. In the world of work, they had relatively low seniority and were unskilled. In categorical terms, fully 22% of those in closing plants had worked for GM for only one or two years. Only 21% from the closing plants worked in skilled trade positions. Racial minorities and females had lower seniority and were less likely than whites and males to be in skilled trades positions. (Almost all of the minority workers were black, and most of the time in the chapters that follow we compare whites with blacks, excluding the 18 racial "other" workers.)

Table 2.1
Demographic Characteristics of Workers
in Closing versus Nonclosing Plants at Wave 1[a]

		Closing (%)	Nonclosing (%)
Characteristics			
Gender			
	Female	26	12
	Male	74	88
Race			
	White	70	79
	Minority	30	21
Seniority			
	Less than 10 years	44	7
	10 to 19 years	37	42
	20 or more years	19	52
Marital Status			
	Married	67	79
	Single	14	5
	Divorced	13	11
	Separated	2	2
	Widowed	1	2
	Cohabitating	3	2
Skill Level			
	Skilled	16	36
	Unskilled	84	64
Averages			
	Age (years)	39.5	44.6
	Education (years)	12.1	12.2
	Seniority (years)	11.9	19.8
	Prior Income (thousands)	38.5	44.6

[a]N = 1,597 workers at Wave 1. Data are in percentages and the column variable, closing/nonclosing plant, is the independent variable. All differences between closing and nonclosing plant workers were statistically significant, except for educational level.

These differences between the closing and nonclosing samples were not entirely unexpected. In fact, the plant closing situation itself may have contributed to the pattern of differences, insofar as high seniority workers -- who were disproportionately older, white males -- were able to transfer out of plants that were scheduled to close.

Interviewing and Response Rates

The initial interviews occurred in late August, September, and October 1987, two to four months before the closing of several General Motors plants in

December 1987. (However, a small proportion of workers from our closing plant sample had already been laid off when we initially interviewed them, as discussed earlier). The same workers were interviewed again at approximately twelve and twenty-four months after the closings. This schedule provided data at points before the actual closings, a short time after the plant closings, and later when major changes in respondents' lives may have occurred.

Wave 1. Wave 1 interviews were conducted in person using trained interviewers. Ten interviewers were UAW retirees previously inexperienced with surveys. They underwent a thorough, week-long training program using guidelines from the University of Michigan's Institute for Social Research. In addition, a commercial research firm, Nordhaus Inc., provided 30 interviewers, all of whom were experienced.

Overall response to the survey was quite favorable. Inability to reach respondents due to lack of correct phone numbers and addresses, rather than refusals, was the most frequent source of nonresponse. It should be noted, however, that some potential respondents were nervous about participating in the survey. Most common were fears that the study was connected with contract negotiations, concerns over confidentiality, and difficulty understanding the purposes of the study. We attempted to address these concerns through careful interviewer training, prior notification letters, interviewer identification, and by alerting local union officials.

Sampling was done randomly and in proportion to plant size within the separate "nonclosing" and "closing" groups. A total sample size of 1,597 completed interviews was obtained: 831 workers from the selected closing plants and 766 from the selected nonclosing plants. Overall, the Wave 1 completion rate was 67% of those contacted. Of course, the sample that results may be biased in unknown ways to the extent that those workers with addresses and telephone numbers we could obtain are different from those for whom we could not obtain this information. We explored the possibility of biases in the sample. The bottom line was reassuring: Workers from closing plants and comparison plants were equally likely to respond (or not respond) to our initial survey, so that comparisons between types of plants are likely to be sound.

Wave 2. Almost all interviews for the second wave were conducted face-to-face, as in the first survey. About 6% of the total interviews in 1988 was, however, conducted by telephone. Many of these were with participants who had moved out of the area, but some were with respondents who indicated that they preferred this mode of interviewing. This procedure proved to be cost-effective, and respondents were pleased with the process. (For these reasons and because preliminary analyses indicated no mode-of-interview effects on the data, we carried out the third wave of the panel study using the telephone as the primary mode of interviewing.)

Workers who had responded to the 1987 first wave survey were the population for the 1988 survey. Various methods were used to locate and interview all of the original 1987 participants. These included, where possible, calling the relative or friend who was identified by the participant as someone who would always know where he/she was, or calling in person at the 1987 address. Original participants who refused to be interviewed in 1988 were also sent follow-up persuasion letters. On the whole, reasons for refusal in 1988 were varied and the bulk of the workers expressed satisfaction with the staff scheduling of interviews.

A very small number of original respondents could not participate because of death (2 people) or incapacitation, including institutionalization (2 people). These were evenly divided between the closing and nonclosing plants, but numbers are too small to do any meaningful assessment of group differences. We include these workers in the totals for "nonrespondents" discussed below.

Overall, the 1988 response rate was a robust 81% (1,288 workers). Of these, 651 (50.5%) came from closing plants and 637 (49.5%) from nonclosing plants. The closing plant response rate was 78%, in contrast to the nonclosing rate of 83%; this difference, although not large, was statistically significant. Overall, the participants were primarily male (81%), white (74%), and married (73%). As in the first wave, closing plant workers were more likely than their nonclosing counterparts to be nonwhite, female, and unmarried.

Wave 3. The 1989 survey sought to reinterview respondents from the 1988 survey. Of the 1,288 respondents from the Wave 2 survey, 1,136 (88%) were reinterviewed in 1989. The sample included 562 workers from closing plants and 574 from nonclosing plants.

Nonresponse

In a panel survey — nonresponse to the second and subsequent waves must be assessed to control for bias. We examined this issue by performing an analysis of respondents and nonrespondents to Waves 2 and 3.

Table 2.2 reports demographic information from Wave 1 regarding Wave 2 nonresponse and from Wave 2 regarding Wave 3 nonresponse. If nonrespondents to the surveys systematically differ from respondents, over time the panel becomes progressively less representative of the population in question. In this case, there were significant differences between respondents and nonrespondents at Waves 2 and 3, as the table summarizes. In both later waves of the survey, closing plant workers were disproportionately represented among the nonrespondents (by a small but significant margin). In Wave 2, nonrespondents were also more likely to have low seniority. And in Wave 3, nonrespondents were disproportionately black and low in education. In addition, Wave 2 nonrespondents were likely to have reported more symptoms of anxiety and depression in Wave 1. Finally, at the bottom of the table, we see that nonrespondents at Wave 2 also scored higher on depression and anxiety at Wave 1.

Table 2.2
Characteristics of Respondents and Nonrespondents[a]

	Wave 2		Wave 3	
	Respondent N = (1,288)	Nonrespondent (309)	Respondent (1,136)	Nonrespondent (152)
Plant Status				
(% closing)	50.5	58.3[b]	49.5	58.6[b]
Gender				
(% female)	19.4	19.7	19.5	19.1
Race				
(% minority)	24.9	28.8	22.9	40.1[b]
Marital Status				
(% married)	73.7	69.9	74.2	69.7
Age				
(years)	42.2	41.0	42.2	42.2
Education				
(years)	12.2	12.2	12.2	11.9[b]
Seniority				
(years)	15.9	14.6[b]	16.0	15.3
Own prior income				
(thousands)	41.0	39.9	41.1	40.1
Depression	1.53	1.61[b]	1.53	1.55
Anxiety	1.43	1.51[b]	1.40	1.44

[a]The column variable, response/nonresponse, is treated as the independent variable in percentages. Demographic and seniority data come from Wave 1.
[b]Respondent-nonrespondent difference significant at p < .05.

Overall, we conclude from this analysis that each difference between the responding and the nonresponding group is likely to make our estimates of hardship and distress relatively conservative. The groups who differentially failed to respond were relatively high-hardship and/or high–distress groups, so the findings may provide *underestimates* of the extent of hardship and distress usually associated with plant closing.

Table 2.3 presents descriptive data for the sociodemographic variables used in the study. Because we often utilize the data for Wave 3 in our analyses, the data presented in the table are for Wave 3.

Now it is time to turn to an overview of the measures used in the study. Items that are used throughout the book are discussed here, whereas measures specific to a particular chapter are given in each later chapter, as the findings are discussed.

Table 2.3
Descriptive Statistics for Demographic Variables

Variable	Minimum	Maximum	Mean	standard deviation	N^a
Number times unemployed	0	3	.53	.82	1,047
Seniority (years)	1	41	15.64	8.88	1,042
Age (years)	21	66	41.78	9.46	1,043
Education (years)	5	16	12.30	1.67	1,046
Prior income (thousands)	5	80	41.19	11.88	1,008
Black (proportion)	0	1	.22	.41	1,047
Female (proportion)	0	1	.19	.39	1,047
Married (proportion)	0	1	.74	.44	1,042

^{a}N = respondents who provided data at all waves, were white or black and had not retired by the second or third wave of the survey.

THE SURVEY QUESTIONS

Wave 1

We developed a questionnaire structured for use in one-hour personal interviews. Questionnaire development was a team effort involving input from members expert in health, psychological, social, and economic areas. Issues covered included the workers' physical health status, psychological well-being, employment and training history and plans, social networks and support systems, family stress and lifestyles, and financial status. Several items were developed from existing questions well established for use in social surveys; others were specifically developed for this study. As part of the questionnaire development and testing, we obtained input on the employment and training items from officials of local unions who participated in the study. As a result, we clarified and revised the wording of several items before conducting the survey. We also used the first week of interviewing as a pretest period, allowing for revisions after testing the questionnaire.

Sections in the questionnaire pertaining to psychological measures, mastery and coping, social support, and life events were adapted from sociopsychological work in these areas. The life events checklist is a modified version of the PERI Life Events Scale (Dohrenwend et al., 1978). This checklist includes negative and neutral events but does not include positive events. It also includes questions concerning the spouse and significant others. Items pertaining to social support were chosen to measure social contacts, organizational membership, and the availability of a confidant. The social support items were derived from work by House, Umberson, & Landis (1988) and Veroff, Douvan, & Kulka (1981).

Several other sections in the questionnaire pertain to nonpsychological measures. These sections include items on employment and training, financial coping and financial status, reactions to the plant closing, physical health, and demographic characteristics. Financial coping questions were adapted from the Employment, Health, and Well-Being Survey by Caplan, Vinokur, Price, & Van Ryn (1989), although substantial alterations were made. Several of the other financial items, as well as items pertaining to employment and training, were developed from union materials. Items on reactions to the plant closing, physical health items, and demographic items were developed by the project team, based upon standard questions used in social surveys.

Second and Third Wave Questionnaires

The second wave questionnaire, like the first, was designed to be used in a one-hour personal interview. Many of the questions were identical to those used in the first wave. The most important additions and modifications to the instrument involved employment status and history. Accurately tracking the employment history of the workers required certain variations in question wording by the time of the second survey. For example, workers in both closing and nonclosing plants might be employed or unemployed; might be looking for alternative employment whether or not they were working; and if unemployed and not looking, might be either permanently or only temporarily out of the workforce. Our questions about employment were, therefore, arranged into seven alternative sections: in the closing plants, sections for workers who were (1) still employed at GM, (2) reemployed elsewhere, (3) looking for work, and (4) at least currently out of the workforce; and in the nonclosing plants, sections for workers who were (5) employed, (6) looking for work, or (7) out of the workforce. We were particularly interested in reemployment and looking for work among the closing plant workers. The survey included detailed questions about the ways the new employment was obtained and about job searches.

Most questions about such topics as health, mental health, drug and alcohol use, and family stress or social support were identical to those in the first wave survey. One change involved closing plant interviews. In the first wave, these had included some questions about coping strategies and about whom the workers blamed for their circumstances; these were not repeated in the second wave. Instead, second wave data included different, but related measures of the worker's sense of mastery (Pearlin et al., 1981) and self-esteem (Rosenberg, 1979).

The Wave 3 interview was essentially the same as in Wave 2, except that mastery and self-esteem scales were asked of all workers.

Measures

Some measures are used throughout the book, and these are discussed here. Measures used that are specific only to a particular chapter are generally discussed in that chapter.

Mental Distress. To measure mental health problems that occur when plants close, we used a checklist in which workers told us how frequently in the past month they had experienced a variety of symptoms. Each survey included a series of 33 items about workers' "problems and complaints" — symptoms of distressed mental health from versions of the HSCL–90 (the Hopkins Symptom Check List (Derogatis, Lipman, Rickels, Uhlenhuth, & Covi, 1974). We averaged answers into four scales to assess particular emotional complaints, depression, anxiety, somaticization, and hostility. The higher the score, the more often the worker reported feeling symptoms. Response choices ranged from 1 = "not at all" to 5 = "a great deal" in the past 30 days.

Depression refers to standard symptoms of clinical depression. Examples of the 12 depression items include "loss of sexual interest or pleasure," "feeling blue," and "thoughts of ending your life." One depression item ("trouble getting to sleep or staying asleep") came from Pearlin et al. (1981). *Anxiety* refers to clinical symptoms of high manifest anxiety. The five scale items include "nervousness" and "trembling." *Somaticization* refers to distress arising from bodily sources (psychosomatic complaints). Samples of the seven items include "headache" and "pains in the chest." *Hostility* refers to feelings of anger and destructive behavior. The four items included "feeling easily annoyed or irritated" and "temper outbursts that you could not control." Each mental health scale was highly reliable at all waves of the study. For somaticization, Cronbach's alpha was .81, .94, and .93 across the three surveys; for anxiety, the corresponding figures were .75, .86, and .87; for hostility, the figures were .76, .76, and .68; and for depression, alpha was .90, .98, and .98. These measures were also highly intercorrelated at each point. At Wave 1, correlations (r) were as follows: depression–anxiety, .82; depression–somatization, .74; depression–hostility, .83; hostility–somatization, .66; hostility–anxiety, .72 and anxiety–somatization, .74; . At Wave 2, corresponding r's were .76, .63, .81, .56, .69, and .69; and at Wave 3 the corresponding r's were .77, .67, .78, .54, .67, and .65. All were highly significant.

The previous literature led us to believe that depression and anxiety would be the most important effects of experiencing plant closure (or its attendant job loss). Further, anxiety should be a kind of leading indicator and depression a lagging indicator; anxiety comes to a head early on in an unemployment experience, distress in general may peak early, and depression may be relatively long–lasting (Cobb & Kasl, 1977; Perrucci et al., 1988). These findings make common sense. Anxiety is diffuse fear. Depression is diffuse despair. We fear what we do not know. We lose hope after we come to know it. Therefore, we may find a kind of flow, a dynamic response to plant closing, in which the balance tips from fear to despair and then, perhaps, back again to some sort of everyday balance.

Somatization, relative to these two other measures, operates as a control variable. Relatively weak relationships, if any, between somatic symptoms and unemployment appear in the literature (e.g., Kessler et al., 1988). Thus we expected somatic complaints to be linked to such factors as the respondent's demographic characteristics, but relatively invariant over time and unresponsive to changes in employment status. We found few effects of somaticization in our study. Finally, although we did think that hostility symptoms would be increased by unemployment, we found a minimal and insignificant relationship. For this reason, we include hostility data only where we did find a significant impact: in relation to men's military and combat experience (see Chapter Seven).

Self-Concept Measures. The self–concept measures used here were the Pearlin et al. (1981) mastery scale and the Rosenberg (1965, 1979) self–esteem scale. In addition to the fact that these are widely used and respected measures, there is a further advantage in the fact that the "stress process", as initially analyzed by Pearlin et al. (1981), featured not only these two theoretical constructs, but also these particular measures.

The Pearlin et al. (1981) mastery scale consists of seven items on a 1–4 scale ("strongly agree" to "strongly disagree"). Five of the seven are worded so that agreement signifies low mastery, such as "I have little control over the things that happen to me" or "There is really no way I can solve the problems I have." In two cases, agreement signifies high mastery ("I can do just about anything I set my mind to" and "What happens to me in the future depends mostly on me"). For scale construction, the five agreement–low mastery items were reverse scored, so that a high score always meant high mastery. Then the mean of the seven items was calculated.

The Rosenberg self–esteem scale includes 10 items on a 1–4 scale (again, "strongly agree" to "strongly disagree"). Five are worded so that agreement indicates high self–esteem, and five low. Items for which agreement indicates high self–esteem include "I take a positive attitude toward myself" and "On the whole, I am satisfied with myself." Items in which agreement indicates low self–esteem include, "All in all, I am inclined to feel that I am a failure" and "I certainly feel useless at times." We reverse the scores of the latter type of item so that a high score always stands for high self–esteem. Then we calculate the mean of responses. We use means, so that the highest score obtainable is a 4.0 and the lowest a 1.0.

To establish the appropriateness of treating each set of items as a unitary scale, we also checked each scale's structure by factor analyzing the items. This is of particular interest in the case of the Rosenberg self–esteem scale, because some researchers find that the positive and negative items load on different factors (self–enhancement and self–denigration; e.g., Owens, 1993). In these data, a simple, single–factor solution was optimal for both mastery and self–esteem. Mastery and self–esteem were highly correlated, not surprisingly. At Wave 2, when only the closing plant workers were asked these questions, mastery and self–esteem correlated .61 (p < .0001); similarly, as of Wave 3 the correlation was .56 for the entire sample. Clearly the overlap between these concepts is substantial; at each wave of the survey, they correlate with one another more highly than either one correlates with itself over time.

Measuring Negative Life Events. In each survey, interviewers asked the workers about whether a series of events had happened to them "in the last twelve months." The list was drawn from a standard life events checklist by Dohrenwend et al. (1978). Following, we divide these into two broad categories, primary and secondary stressors (Pearlin, 1989). A primary stressor is an independent source of stress that may help to tip the balance between health and illness, happiness and distress. A secondary stressor is not necessarily any less important or any smaller than a primary one, but it follows from or results from a primary stressor.

Within primary stressors, we initially distinguished among four categories of events:

1. broken ties, referring to the breaking off of a love relationship;
2. loss of loved ones, referring to loss of a loved one by death;
3. other crises, referring to a variety of serious crises that could occur to the self (such as being in an accident or having one's house burn down). 4. The fourth group of stressors, of course, was secondary events, which we argue on logical grounds are likely to be consequences of plant closing or unemployment (e.g., having to move).

These various stressors are concrete and are best grasped by imagining the concrete situations in which they leave people. It is difficult indeed to imagine what "the last twelve months" might have been like for the worker who answered "yes" to many, or even several, of the events listed below. Arranged by category (and also roughly by the order of their presentation), the events were as follows:

1. Broken ties
   Engagement broken or love affair ended
   Marital separation
   Divorced
2. Loved ones lost
   Spouse/partner died
   Your child died
   Relative (other than partner or child) died
   Close friend died
3. Other crises
   Lost home through fire, flood, or other disaster
   Physically attacked or assaulted
   Burglarized or robbed

A serious accident or injury
A serious accident started or got worse
4. Women also could suffer four additional events:
An abortion
Miscarriage or still birth
Found out you cannot have children
Started menopause

Secondary events and their rationale. We designated some events as secondary to be as careful as possible about making such assertions as: "Plant closings cause other tragedies," or "The loss of a job causes other things in a person's life to unravel." In some cases, the linkage between the two may not be especially meaningful. There may be such a close logical or psychological connection that what we really have isn't so much two separate events as a succession of acts in a single unfolding tragedy. Therefore, we separated out seven events that we felt confident would be affected by plant closing or by unemployment. Two of these were financial, involving repossession of belongings and general financial or property loss. Five of them referred to persons moving in or out of the worker's home or to the worker's move to a worse neighborhood, a new area, or a new state. (It seemed highly likely that one response to job loss, for example, would be moving to find work.)

In addition, for married workers and those living with someone, these life events questions were followed by five items about the person's spouse or partner (or, in the case of men, nine items, including the same four events that were listed above for female workers). And for workers with children under age 18, we asked a set of six questions about negative events in the children's lives.

Scaling. Life events researchers either treat these events using some kind of weighting procedure (so that worse happenings are weighted more heavily) or they simply add them up. Summing of events is certainly the simplest procedure, and for many purposes, weighted measures do not perform any better (Dohrenwend & Dohrenwend, 1981). For each of the four types of events—broken ties, loss of loved one, other crises, and secondary events—we constructed a sum, so that each worker's score could theoretically run from zero to the total number of events in that category. For each wave of the survey, we also constructed an index of 24 nonfinancial, potentially negative, life events (this summary measure is generally referred to simply as "negative life events" in the tables).

Social Support. We measured six potential sources of social support: organized athletic activity; union membership and degree of participation; membership and degree of activity in clubs and organizations; frequency of attending religious services; frequency of getting together with neighbors, friends, or relatives; and having or not having others to confide in. Our measure of having a confidant is based on a question which read, "Is there anyone in your life with whom you have a close and confiding relationship, with whom you can share your most private feelings?" Virtually everyone at every wave of the survey had at least one such someone. We asked follow–up questions about who this person was, including the person's relationship to the worker. The interviewers continued to probe for up to four of these people in whom the worker might confide. For the other measures of support, we asked about the frequency of participation in an activity. Each time we asked about it, activity level had the same six categories: "more than once a week, once a week, two or three times a month, about once a month, less than once a month, or never." For the questions on organized athletic activities; union activities and clubs and organizations other than a union, we converted responses into seven–category variables, assigning a value of 1 to not a member, then values of 2 through 7 to the different levels of activity among members. For the other two questions, frequency of getting together with friends and neighbors, and frequency of attending religious services, a 1 through 6 scale was used, because we did not assign a value for "not a member."

Family Conflict. We used several measures to ascertain the level of family conflict. First, four questions dealt with the way workers and their spouses got along during the previous 12 months:

How often did you and your partner quarrel?
How often did you and your partner get on each other's nerves?
How often did you insult or scream at each other?
How often did you push or hit each other?

Choices of answers were given in terms of time periods rather than in more evaluative terms (such as "often" or "rarely") in an attempt to lessen the tendency of workers to give socially desirable answers. Choices were "never, once a month, a few times a month, weekly, or a few times a week."

A parallel set of questions was asked of workers who had children. In the past 12 months,

How often do you and your child(ren) have unpleasant arguments with one another?
How often do you and your child(ren) get on each other's nerves?
How often do you lose control of your temper when dealing with your children?
How often do you or your partner hit, slap, or spank your child(ren)?

Again the choices were "never, once a month, a few times a month, weekly, or a few times a week."We assigned a value of 1 for an answer of "never" and a 5 for an answer of "a few times a week," so that a high score indicates high conflict. For both the spouse and child, only the first three of the questions listed above are averaged together in this summary because almost no workers admitted to pushing or hitting a spouse, and relatively few said they hit, slapped, or spanked children. As a result, the answers to the hitting questions simply did not have enough variance to scale with other answers about family conflict. Therefore, both measures of spouse conflict and child conflict use the three measures for each subject, excluding hitting. Frequency of conflict (from very often to never) was averaged across items. Scores range from 3 to 15 for each measure. Although we exclude analysis of hitting spouse, the item for child hitting is examined separately, because there was some variability in responses.

There is one important caveat to keep in mind when we discuss family stress: Our data are obtained from the workers themselves, not from their wives and husbands and children. Insofar as workers give answers from their own perspective, these answers may differ from what their spouse or child would say. And as the emotional content of a question rises, answers to it probably become more self–defensive or self–justifying. We might find more instances of serious quarreling (such as hitting of the partner or spouse) if we were able to ask that person directly. Therefore, answers about family conflict should not be taken as literal, accurate, reports of conflict. What such answers do reflect is *what workers thought was the emotional health of the home, or what they were willing to tell us about it.*

A large research literature exists about the accuracy of "proxy reporting," that is, offering answers about the opinions, behaviors, or characteristics of another person. Proxy reports are essential in some areas, such as research on the health and welfare of children. Proxy reporting about adults is often done to save money or time (as in this study) or to help in assessing a particularly sensitive issue such as problem drinking. The answers of a "proxy" may be more trustworthy than a person's own where such issues are concerned. For example, a husband's two beers a night may turn into three, or four, or six as viewed by the wife. A growing body of data also pertains to the specific issue of the convergence or divergence of answers by husbands and wives about problems or conflicts. Divergences exist over such issues as when they were married or how many rooms are in the house, but the divergences are predictably more serious and more systematic in sensitive areas. Stress and conflict are among the most troublesome sensitive issues to investigate because they are interactive: they involve and may implicate the proxy just as much as the "actor." Every reality gets distorted by the particular lens through which it is seen.

In sum, we wish we knew what the husbands, wives or partners of these workers would have said about the family's emotional atmosphere. What we have here is the presumably self–protective or even self–serving answers of one part of the puzzle of conflict. Another study will have to assess the accuracy of using proxies for family stress as we do here.

Financial Hardship. Each survey asked a variety of questions about financial hardships during the preceding months or year. At each wave of the survey, workers were asked the extent to which they had done a number of things that indicate financial difficulty. First, they were asked a series of eight items about actions they may have taken in the previous 12 months. These items were cut back purchases, decided not to buy planned purchase, drawn more heavily from savings than usual, postponed nonemergency medical or dental care because of cost, borrowed money to help pay bills, used credit cards or installment plans more than usual, missed mortgage or rent payments, and missed other payments. Workers were asked to rate whether they did each action "a great deal," "quite a bit," "some," "little," or "not at all." We refer to this group of items as minor hardships. Then, workers were asked a series of eight more questions regarding what we considered to be more extreme steps. These items were used Medicare/Medicaid, used food stamps, used public assistance, used rent/heat subsidy, moved to lower payments, and pawned or sold items. Answers were simply yes/no questions, on the theory that doing them at all was indicative of financial trouble. We refer to these items as major hardships. Another four–part question asked about difficulty in obtaining certain basics (food, medical care, clothing, and leisure activities). In each case, the workers were offered four possible responses: "never," "once in a while," "fairly often," or "very often." Finally, an item we refer to as bills asked about overall difficulty in paying bills. (Options included "extremely difficult or impossible," "very difficult," "somewhat difficult," "slightly difficult," and "not at all difficult.")

For some workers—those who had children between the ages of five and twenty–two (school or college aged), an additional set of questions asked whether or not any of their children had to cut back, stop, or not begin various activities due to the family's finances. Two questions regarding employment and college education were also asked about older children. All questions about children were simple yes/no choices.

Whether the issue was inability to pay bills, difficulty in feeding and clothing the family, scrimping on medical care, or engaging in a series of behaviors reflective of financial difficulties (such as delayed bill paying, running up credit card bills, missing mortgage payments, or accepting public assistance), females reported significantly higher evidence of hardship than males at all waves of the study; so did blacks in comparison to whites. For present purposes, we use a summary indicator of the financial hardships reported in Wave 3 as having occurred during the previous year. This summary was created by transforming three measures—minor financial hardships, difficulty in obtaining the basics, and difficulty in paying bills—into percentile scores and averaging them. Therefore, the measure ranges from 0 to 100, and high scores indicate greater hardship.

Table 2.3 presents descriptive statistics for demographic variables used throughout most of the book; these data are provided here so that the reader can gain some perspective of the study.

Supplementing the Panel Study

In the summer of 1991, four and a half years after the plants closed, we obtained a limited amount of additional data. The panel surveys had given us the quantitative data, but the time constraints in these large–scale surveys did not give us the freedom to let the workers speak for themselves about the closings and more fully about their lives. We decided to try a more intensive, open–ended interview with a small number of workers to flesh out the picture.

We selected closing plant workers who were at two extremes of depression: 15 who never reported any symptoms versus 15 who were in the top 10% of scorers at all three interviews. Overall, by these criteria, 22 closing plant workers were consistently high, and 62 were consistently low in depression ("undepressed") across the three surveys. Interviews by telephone lasted approximately 45 minutes. Among the interviewees, 34% of the nondepressed and 54% of the highly depressed were female; and 34% of the low depression and 40% of the high depression group were black.

These interviews were used as a source of texture to enrich the quantitative findings; they are the source of the quotes in the book. To smooth the flow of remarks in their written form, we have sometimes combined sentences or linked fragmentary remarks into sentences. Care was taken to avoid any disturbance of the original meaning.

OVERVIEW

This is a study of the way the 1987 GM plant closings affected the personal, familial, and work lives of those who once worked in those plants. This chapter has outlined and described some of the potential consequences of a plant closing and how we went about studying them. We rely mainly on large–scale panel surveys, as described in this chapter, with supplemental information from follow–up interviews with workers who were extreme cases with regard to depression in the large–scale surveys. The chapter has concentrated on the mechanics of the research: the where, who, and how. The chapters that follow tell about the what, what we found out, and a bit about the why, why it occurred, in this particular type and time and occasion for stress.

The bottom line of a plant closing is stress. When the plant doors shut, lives constrict. Some workers lose their jobs. Other workers no longer have good jobs. Still others manage to hang on to the status quo but with reduced confidence about the future for themselves or their children. The fact of a job and the quality of that job are linked to a host of financial, psychological, and physical health consequences. Our surveys have asked about what happens in a plant closing, to whom it happens, and what it means to those who must live through it. The coming chapters will document that workers whose plants close suffer job losses, financial hardships, symptoms of poor mental health, and marital strains.

3

Unemployment and Reemployment

After the plant closing, I went to school for computers through the Human Resource Center. My wife went to work, but we have children. So between my schooling and her job, we did what we could to keep the house together. After I graduated from school in computer drafting, I couldn't find a job. Well, I ended up working as a retail clerk in warehousing. I went from $14.00 to $6.80, and now I am at $9.00—the top of my labor grade. This has an effect on things at home. It is stressful. We were young and upgrading our lifestyle and then lost it all. The family is just not the same. It isn't the home it was.
—a closing plant worker

I was unemployed for a long time and things were getting tougher at home. I got the chance to take a transfer to another facility several states away. I had to take it and leave my family behind in Michigan...It is not so easy to be so far from home. But I wouldn't move my family here. I own a house in Michigan and my kids are in school there. I can't just uproot them and bring them here. I don't know if it would work out. So, every few weeks or so, some of us carpool and head back for two days. I should be there with my family . . . but what can I do?
—a closing plant worker

When people think of a plant closing, what comes to mind first is loss of jobs. Second, we tend to reflect on the workers' limited chances to gain new jobs of any quality. When the employer is a giant like GM, however, even job loss is not so necessary or so automatic as it might at first seem. Unlike small companies, GM can boast other plants to which workers might be sent and other jobs they might be able to fill. Therefore, a first question in the case of plant closings by an industrial giant is deceptively simple: Did workers lose jobs, and if so, how many? Did the losers regain jobs, and if so, where? We turn to these facts next. Because of their general importance in the sociological literature and their role in our own data, we pay special attention here to how blacks and women fared, in comparison to their white, male counterparts.

First, it is important to clarify terms. For the most part, this chapter uses the terms "unemployed" or "not employed" in their most general sense to include all those who are not working (even retired workers). We do so because at Wave 1, there were no retired workers to enumerate. Later chapters often delete retirees from the analyses, especially when addressing theoretical issues regarding the stress of unemployment. The text or accompanying footnotes always indicate upon which cases a given analysis focuses.

TRENDS IN JOBS

When we first talked to them in August through October 1987, the large majority of workers from both closing and nonclosing plants were employed. Yet Chapter Two has already noted that permanent layoffs were occurring well before the actual plant closures and even before interviewing began. At the time of the Wave 1 survey, 24% of the 832 closing plant workers were already unemployed. In the nonclosing plants, no workers were unemployed. Statistically, the difference between closing and nonclosing plant workers was highly significant. The overall employment picture for a worker whose plant closed changed drastically and for the worse with plant closure. One and two years after the fact, striking differences remained in workers' likelihood of being employed and of being satisfied with that employment, depending on whether they started out in a closing or a non-closing plant. At Wave 2, one year after closure, 50% of the closing plant workers were not employed, in contrast to 10% of workers in nonclosing plants. At Wave 3, two years after closure, 35% of closing plant workers were still not employed, compared with 9% of their nonclosing counterparts.

One rough–and–ready way to assess the cumulative impact of having or not having a job is simply to tally how many times the worker did or didn't have one. Such a summary score does not distinguish such refinements as whether the worker is even currently employed or not (if the worker's score is zero or three instances of unemployment, this can be inferred; otherwise, for scores of one or two unemployment periods, it cannot). However, our analyses using multiple measures of unemployment (occurrence, frequency, and duration) indicate that at least in these data, little is lost by using a summary like this. And much is gained in the ability to depict trends via figures and graphs. Throughout the book, when we use this summary measure, number of times unemployed, we often indicate how alternative measures of unemployment performed, if there is any critical difference.

Using the summary measure of number of times unemployed, how many times did each worker tell the interviewer that he or she was not employed across the three waves of surveys? None, one, two, or three? The answer is very different for a worker whose plant closed and a worker whose plant did not.

Figure 3.1 summarizes patterns of joblessness across surveys in terms of whether the workers came from closing or nonclosing plants. Some results are predictable. Because only employed workers from nonclosing plants were initially interviewed, the category "not employed all three times" has no workers from plants that did not close. But there is also a consistent difference everywhere else in Figure 3.1. Workers from nonclosing plants were far more likely to be steadily employed. Closing plant workers were more likely to have fallen out of the labor force, whether this was once, twice, or three times.

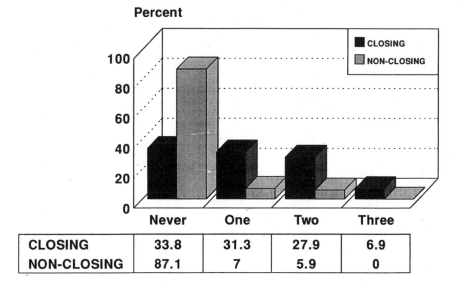

	Never	One	Two	Three
CLOSING	33.8	31.3	27.9	6.9
NON-CLOSING	87.1	7	5.9	0

Figure 3.1. Differences between closing and nonclosing plant workers in the number of times without a job during the panel study.

REEMPLOYMENT

There are several issues to be considered concerning the question of the way people get new jobs:

1. What are the realities of the local and larger labor market? Is it possible or plausible that workers will get new jobs quickly? That they will get good jobs? That they will find themselves able to do so without moving out of town, out of state, or even out of the region?
2. What do workers themselves want to do?
3. What do they realistically expect will happen?
4. How do they try to make jobs happen?
5. Do the wants, expectations, and efforts translate into jobs? What kind of jobs? Where?
6. Do we have any evidence of differences in who is laid off and who gets to return to GM: in particular, any linkage to race or to gender? These comparisons need to be made both overall, and taking seniority into account; the former provides the global picture of demographic difference, and the latter tells us whether this difference can be accounted for by the lower seniority of some groups.

We address each of these six issues in turn.

The Local Labor Market. The local labor market offered these workers some hope, but it was not what they would ideally want. Although the likelihood of finding a job was reasonable, the likelihood of finding a job with anywhere near the same pay and benefits was virtually nonexistent. Although we consider this reality later in the chapter, the quotes from the workers at the beginning of the chapter amply illustrate the issues. Workers had to move out of town to get a job with G.M. or another auto company to get the same type of job with the same pay and benefits. The options in town were considerably less. Because most workers who lost their jobs did not move out of the Detroit and Flint areas, the remainder of this chapter shows in stark detail the inability to find jobs like those they lost.

Workers' Definitions of Their Position in the Labor Market. By the time we talked to them one and two years after the plant closings, workers could be in a variety of employment or unemployment situations. Whether originally in a closing or a nonclosing plant, a worker might be (1) still working for GM, or instead, working for another employer. If the job was new, the worker might be (2) basically satisfied with the new job -- considering it a permanent one -- or might be (3) employed but still looking for better work. Among workers who were not employed, we found four self-defined categories. Some were in the classical position of being (4) unemployed and looking for work. Others were (5) unemployed, but at least temporarily not actively looking for work. Still others had become discouraged and considered themselves (6) out of the work force. Finally, some had (7) retired. These categories reflect both workers' objective circumstances and their intentions, plans, or decisions about what, if anything, to do to alter those circumstances. Thus, it may be helpful to take a more fine–tuned look at the "employed" versus "not employed," as seen through the workers' eyes.

Table 3.1 shows the distribution of these seven employment statuses at Wave 2, one year after closure, and at Wave 3, two years after. Because essentially none of the nonclosing plant workers and relatively few closing plant workers were doing part–time work, we have combined full–time and part–time workers. (Many part–timers were dissatisfied with the work, putting them in category 3 of the scheme outlined above.)

To begin with, Table 3.1 shows that those who started out in nonclosing plants were overwhelmingly employed at GM one and two years later. Only small percentages described themselves as being in any other situation. In Wave 2, some nonclosing plant workers -- less than 10% -- were looking for work or were unemployed but not actively looking. By Wave 3, most of these had found jobs that they considered permanent with other employers. Overall, for those who started out in the nonclosing plants, "work" basically means stable employment with the same employer.

Workers from closing plants faced a very different reality. By Wave 2, only 24% of them still worked at GM, a figure that dropped to 18% in the following year. At Wave 2, half of all closing plant workers were not employed and 9% of those who had jobs wanted to change them. In addition, fully 29% of the closing plant workers were unemployed and looking for work. This picture improved by Wave 3 but remained drastically different from that for nonclosing plant workers. Although two-thirds had jobs by the third survey, 14% of closing plant workers

Table 3.1

Employment Status — Closing versus Nonclosing Plants

(Percent of Respondents)[a]

Employment status	Wave 2		Wave 3	
	Closing N = 651	Nonclosing 637	Closing 532	Nonclosing 569
Work at GM	24.1	86.0	18.2	84.4
New job	16.6	1.4	34.5	7.0
Job but looking	9.1	1.7	14.3	1.2
Unemployed looking	29.0	4.1	18.4	1.9
Unemployed temporarily	17.1	3.1	9.8	2.6
Out of workforce	1.2	.2	1.1	.4
Retired	2.9	3.5	2.6	2.5

[a]Differences between closing and nonclosing plants for both years are significant at p < .01 using chi-square test.

were dissatisfied and seeking to change those jobs. This figure is about 12 times greater than the comparable figure for workers in nonclosing plants.

In later chapters we will probe further into questions of the meaning of employment versus unemployment for these workers. Later chapters will probe the psychological implications of being in the various self–defined job statuses for the worker's levels of depression/ sense of mastery, self–esteem. Later in this chapter we will offer more details of the working conditions, pay, and the like that may account for the reasons that some workers are satisfied and others are not. For present purposes, Table 3.1 simply fleshes out the simple dichotomy, employed–unemployed; it illustrates that stark differences in life courses and life chances opened up between workers as a function of their plant being closed or spared.

New Jobs: Expectations. Because very few workers were in a position to retire, most had to face the realities of securing employment elsewhere. We asked workers a series of questions about what they thought their job search would be like. Then, for workers who had become reemployed, we asked about the characteristics of their new jobs. Now we can match the expectations to the realities.

In Wave 1 we asked workers a series of questions about the jobs for which they would be looking.

Table 3.2 summarizes their responses concerning how difficult they thought it would be to find a job (1) that paid at least the same wages as the job they had before plant closure, (2) that had the same benefits, and (3) that had working conditions at least as pleasant. A great majority of workers thought it would be impossible or difficult to match their GM wages and benefits. In contrast, most workers felt it would hardly be difficult to match the working conditions of their GM job. (We can infer that they found these conditions less appealing, at least relatively speaking, than they found their pay or benefits to be.)

Table 3.2
Expectations About Wages, Benefits, and Working Conditions

Ability to obtain a job with	Same wages %	Same benefits %	Pleasant Working conditions %
Impossible	40	41	12
Very difficult	41	41	17
Somewhat difficult	15	14	26
Not at all difficult	5	5	44

Table 3.3 shows what closing plant workers were expecting—or willing—to go through to get and keep these new, less attractive jobs. A small proportion thought they would definitely have to move, either within Michigan or outside the state. In contrast, a majority thought they would definitely or very likely need retraining. Workers were willing to make long commutes to these new jobs. More than a third claimed that they would commute 50 miles or more each way. And the minimum hourly wage that closing plant workers said they would accept was more than $3.00 less than what they were currently making (an average of $9.85, as opposed to their current $13.13).

What workers envisioned as they faced the closing of the plants is evident. Given the prospect, or at least the possibility, of unemployment, workers held diminished expectations about future jobs. These numbers testify to a combination of eagerness to work, a sense of urgency about finding work, and pessimism about the type of work to be found. Objectively, the UAW contract provided numerous guarantees, but the psychological reality for these workers probably included a sense of doors closing on more than one job or one plant.

The Job Search Process. We asked a series of questions about the job search process: where workers looked for jobs, whether help was received from the union or GM in looking for a new job, and whether workers had to move to secure employment.

Table 3.4 presents data on how workers went about looking for new jobs. The table presents data for closing plant workers only. The groups are divided into closing plant workers who were employed and not looking for other jobs, closing plant workers who were employed but actively looking for other jobs, and closing

Table 3.3
Expectations about Moving, Retraining, Wages, and Commute

New job will require:	Move inside Michigan %	Move outside Michigan %	Retraining %
Definitely	9	6	37
Very Likely	14	12	20
Somewhat Likely	30	29	20
Not At All Likely	48	53	24

Acceptable wage		Maximum commute (one way):	
Less than $3.35	1	Under 20 miles	10
3.36 to 5.00	4	20 to 29	22
5.01 to 9.99	39	30 to 39	21
10.00 to 14.99	49	40 to 49	11
15.00 to 19.99	7	50 to 74	34
20.00 or more	1	75 plus	2

plant workers who were not employed. In general, most workers look at want ads, contact potential employers, and ask friends and others in seeking new jobs. It is significant that only a small portion of workers got job leads from GM or the UAW. Comparing across the groups of workers, we see there is much similarity between the people who describe themselves as looking for work, whether or not they are employed. The percentages tend to be lower by year three, but the difference is not a dramatic one.

Table 3.4
Actions Taken During Job Search

% yes	Closing (Working)	Wave 2 Closing (Looking–employed)	Closing (Looking– not employed)
Want ads	78.6	91.5	95.2
Employment Agency	24.3	30.5	28.2
Ask friends	82.5	89.8	89.3
Ask others	72.8	88.1	88.8
Public employment agency	62.1	71.2	71.3
Contact potential employers	77.7	91.5	83.5
Seek counseling	44.1	40.7	45.7
Get leads from GM	13.6	20.3	14.4
Get leads from UAW	12.6	20.3	21.8
Use joint training	30.4	31.0	42.2
Informational interviews	35.9	44.1	45.2
N =	103	59	188

% yes	Closing (Working)	Wave 3 Closing (Looking–employed)	Closing (Looking– not employed)
Want ads	73.0	98.7	96.9
Employment Agency	23.3	28.9	20.4
Ask friends	69.8	93.4	86.7
Ask others	67.7	86.8	85.6
Public employment agency	52.9	67.1	78.4
Contact potential employers	68.3	97.4	78.6
Seek counseling	26.5	43.4	40.8
Get leads from GM	13.8	11.8	18.6
Get leads from UAW	20.6	15.8	16.5
Use joint training	26.7	36.5	31.3
Informational interviews	28.7	40.8	42.3
N =	189	76	98

Table 3.5 presents data on the information workers might have received. Most frequently, workers received information about unemployment compensation. A majority of workers received information about tuition assistance and training. By year three, a much smaller portion of workers received information.

Table 3.6 presents data on the use of public agencies by these workers. We expected that many workers would use MESC (the Michigan Employment Security Commission) because this is the office where many must report to receive unemployment compensation. By Wave 2 of our survey, 92% of workers reported going there at some point in the year, whereas the figures had dropped significantly by year three. We were also interested in whether workers would use the various helping agencies available to them. A small number of workers did use these agencies, and workers who were not employed were more likely to do so.

Table 3.5
Percent Saying They Received Information on. . . .

% yes	Closing employed	Year 2 Closing looking– employed	Closing looking–not employed
Continue health benefits	56.9	52.5	58.0
Unemployment and SUB	65.7	72.9	66.7
Tuition assistance	59.4	52.5	56.1
Training programs	54.5	52.5	50.8
Job with GM	27.7	20.7	21.9
Other job	35.0	30.5	23.8
Dealing with stress	31.7	22.0	30.3
Financial assistance	19.0	17.2	17.1
N =	102	59	188

% yes	Closing employed	Year 3 Closing looking– employed	Closing looking–not employed
Continue health benefits	39.2	25.3	42.6
Unemployment and SUB	34.4	25.3	43.1
Tuition assistance	42.3	45.8	56.9
Training programs	37.0	47.0	50.6
Job with GM	21.2	13.3	23.1
Other job	23.3	30.1	28.7
Dealing with stress	15.9	18.1	15.7
Financial assistance	15.9	14.5	13.9
N =	189	83	108

Table 3.6
Use of Public Agencies by Closing Plant Workers

	Year 2		Year 3	
	Not employed	Employed outside GM	Not employed	Employed outside GM
Percentage using				
M.E.S.C.	92.0	92.6	50.0	62.5
Social services	6.2	10.5	5.8	13.1
Soc. Security	4.9	8.1	3.2	13.6
Health Dept.	6.2	3.4	3.2	7.4
Bd. Education	13.0	23.3	13.1	25.1
Legal aid	4.9	6.8	5.8	4.0
Child/family svcs.	3.7	3.0	3.8	3.4
Churches/ synagogue	7.4	11.5	11.9	14.2
Other state job training	3.7	10.2	2.6	6.3
N =	162	295	312	176

Getting the New Job. One initial fear in many minds was that workers and their families would need to uproot themselves to get jobs. Before considering the types and numbers of jobs obtained, we therefore asked where the jobs were.

As Table 3.7 shows, only a small number of workers moved as a result of being laid off. Whatever their quality and quantity, the jobs obtained were primarily a local affair.

Table 3.7
Percentage of Closing Plant Workers Who Moved as a Result of Being Laid Off[a]

	Wave 2		Wave 3	
	employed	Not employed	employed	Not employed
Move elsewhere	7.2 (321)	8.1 (298)	8.6 (362)	9.3 (150)
Necessary to move to find new job	47.8 (23)	16.7 (24)	56.3 (32)	42.9 (16)

[a]N's in parentheses

Next, the quantity and quality of work: We have seen that many workers in closing plants had to deal with unemployment and had to absorb psychologically the possibility that future work would never be the same again. But what about the reality of reemployment? Next, we look at whether the workers' diminished expectations about future jobs were reflected in the jobs they actually landed.

Some closing plant workers were able to remain at GM, either never getting laid off or returning after a period of unemployment. But workers who had to leave GM to find work often had to leave the industrial manufacturing sector. By Wave 2, half of the workers from closing plants who were employed were no longer at GM. Of the workers who had found jobs elsewhere, only 61 had new jobs in industrial manufacturing. Most (99 workers) had found employment in other blue collar or service jobs such as construction, bus driving, working in repair shops of various types, and clerking in stores. The small remainder was self–employed (in such jobs as beautician, house cleaner, and photographer) or worked for a government organization.

Table 3.8 shows the job status of closing and nonclosing plant workers as of Waves 2 and 3 of our study. In both years only a small percentage of the closing plant workers were still employed at GM: about 23% as of Wave 2, dropping to 18% by Wave 3. In contrast, approximately 85% of the nonclosing plant workers were still employed at GM. In Wave 2, 17% of closing plant workers had found new jobs, 29% were unemployed and looking for new jobs, and 17% were unemployed and *not* looking for work. Recall that these are people who say that they will look for a new job in the near future but are not now looking for a new job. A small number of workers had retired or were otherwise out of the workforce. By Wave 3, the situation was very different. Importantly, about twice as many people as in Wave 2 had new jobs. If we add the rows a bit, we see that almost 70% of workers were employed in Wave 3. However, it is still true that more than 18% of workers from the closing plants were unemployed and looking for work, a figure approximately ten times that for nonclosing plant workers. In addition, the fact that about 14% of these closing plant workers in Wave 3 who had a job were still looking for another, indicates at least some level of dissatisfaction with what they had found.

What are the implications of the new mix of jobs for workers' financial well–being? One way of comparing work situations is to look at the combination of pay and benefits available.

Table 3.9 summarizes the picture for Wave 2 and Wave 3, showing that workers who found new jobs were considerably less well off than workers who remained GM employees. In Wave 2, workers who still worked for GM versus those who did not were compared. In Wave 3 the same series of questions was asked only of those workers from the closing plants who had obtained new jobs.

In Table 3.9, there is a marked difference at Wave 2 between workers who found or continued jobs with GM and those who did not. Only about two-thirds of

Table 3.8
Year Two and Three Job Status by Closing vs. Nonclosing Status

	Year 2		Year 3	
	Closing	Nonclosing	Closing	Nonclosing
GM employee	23.1	86.0	18.2	84.4
New job	16.6	1.4	35.5	7.0
Job but looking	9.1	1.7	14.3	1.2
Looking	29.0	4.1	18.4	1.9
Unemployed	17.1	3.1	9.8	2.6
Out of workforce	1.2	0.2	1.1	0.4
Retired	2.9	3.5	2.6	2.5
N	651	637	532	569

those workers who found new jobs in Wave 2 had the same benefits as they had when they were working for GM. Only 66% had dental benefits, 68% had life insurance, and only about 70% had paid vacations. Relative to some jobs, of course, no one would describe such percentages as "only"—but compared to a sure thing, even 70% is "only" 70%. To put it in the negative, roughly a third of the newly employed workers had gained jobs but had lost potentially crucial benefits which had been a routine fact of life when they worked at GM. And losses were not

Table 3.9
Characteristics of Current Job
(Percent of Respondents From Closing Plants)

Benefits	Wave 2		Wave 3
	Working for GM	Working elsewhere	Working elsewhere
	N=53	103	189
Health care	98.1	79.6	90.4
Dental	96.2	66.0	81.3
Eye	96.2	62.1	77.2
Life insurance	98.1	68.9	81.9
Pension plan	98.1	62.7	80.6
Paid vacation	96.2	69.9	89.4
Wages higher than last job	20.8	19.6	18.7
Wages lower than last job	22.6	63.7	47.6
Conditions as good	78.4	85.1	85.7
Needed retraining	25.9	24.3	23.4
Average hourly pay	$14.92	$10.13	$11.13

just personal. For those workers who had families, benefit coverage for their children was also cut.

The change in benefits may be understated by these numbers because it is likely that the benefit coverage with other employers was in fact less comprehensive than that provided in the contract with GM; only detailed questions about such issues as the cost sharing required of the employee, the presence of disability insurance, and the like would have uncovered such finely–tuned differences. In addition, our questions did not specifically include an item about the availability of pensions.

The drop in wages was even more extreme than the loss of benefits, as the bottom portion of the table shows. Well over half (63%) had lower wages in their current jobs than in their old jobs at GM. The vast majority, more than 85%, had also needed retraining to get this lower paying job. The most positive picture of the new employment situation was in fact predicted by the workers at Wave 1. More than half found that their new working conditions to be as pleasant as those at their old job at GM.

In terms of literal dollars earned, the last row of the table shows a large gulf between closing plant workers who did and did not remain at GM. To have to leave GM meant about a one–third loss in pay. What the table does not show is an equally impressive similarity: There was no significant difference between the average hourly wage earned by closing plant workers who stayed at GM and that earned by the nonclosing plant GM workers (both earned about $14.90 per hour).

By Wave 3, the situation for those with new jobs was a bit better, whether it was due to a better mix of new jobs obtained or a better package of benefits becoming available from employers as seniority was gained. But the benefit and wage gaps remained. Workers who no longer worked for GM still missed out on key benefits, and about half of the workers who had new jobs in Wave 3 reported that they received lower wages in their current jobs than at GM. Although the last row shows a somewhat higher hourly wage for these workers than they had made in the previous year, the gap between them and any workers still at GM remained about $5 per hour.

To sum up, the closing of the plants brought two kinds of threats to the financial resources of workers. First, of course, many lost jobs for at least some period of time. Some even lost them before the plants closed. Even two years after the plant closings, many workers remained unemployed. And second, reemployment was a mixed blessing unless the worker was able to get back inside GM. Many had to leave the manufacturing world which had been their work home. A sizeable number had to face the risk of going without some or all of the benefits, such as hospitalization, that cushion the modern worker against medical disaster. And most had to accept lower wages than they had earned at GM. Their Wave 1 responses told us that this is what the workers expected. It is clearly what they got.

Who Got Laid Off? Who Got to Return?

Table 3.10 examines who these workers were, in terms of their demographic characteristics. Comparing the group of closing plant workers, we see that workers who were employed were more likely to be white, male and married. There were few differences between employed and unemployed workers on the other demographic characteristics.

Table 3.11 tells us about the *differential* impact of plant closing on a sampling of outcomes which are of particular importance to later chapters: the workers' levels of depression and anxiety (the remainder of the book), the stress experienced with spouse and children (latter part of Chapter Four), and financial hardships Chapter Six). In the table, we compare three groups of closing plant workers:

Table 3.10
Demographic Profiles by Employment Status
For Workers in Closing versus Nonclosing Plants, Years Two and Three[a]

| | Year 2 | | | |
| | Closing | | Control | |
	EMP[b]	UN[b]	EMP	UN[b]
% white	74.4	66.0	79.4	76.1
% male	81.5	64.0	90.1	63.0
% married	72.6	60.3	82.0	67.4
Age	39.6	39.0	44.1	42.5
Education	12.3	12.0	12.3	12.1
Income	39.9	37.4	43.5	43.1
Seniority	11.7	11.7	19.5	15.4
N =	322	298	565	46

| | Year 3 | | | |
| | Closing | | Control | |
	EMP[b]	UN[b]	EMP	UN[b]
% white	74.3	72.7	80.3	76.9
% male	78.2	64.0	89.4	73.1
% married	69.8	60.0	81.8	73.1
Age	38.9	40.4	43.9	48.3
Education	12.4	11.8	12.4	11.4
Income	39.2	37.3	43.6	43.2
Seniority	11.0	13.6	19.3	20.8
N =	360	149	525	26

[a] Mean values are presented for age, education, income (in thousands) and seniority.
[b] EMP = employed, UN = unemployed.

first, the group of workers who were unemployed at wave two, but employed at wave three; second, workers who were unemployed at both waves; and third, workers who were employed at both waves. (We are leaving out the small group of workers who became unemployed for the first time as of wave three, because they would have had minimal opportunity to obtain reemployment.) In the analyses of covariance we conducted, the cells of the table are adjusted means (controlling for age, sex, race, education, income, and seniority; for whether the worker had a confidant or not; and for the wave one measure of the dependent variable.) The results can be read as referring to the change in hardships, distress, and conflict for these three employment status groups, taking into account their demographic characteristics. A multiple regression analysis which controlled for the preceding variables and used dummy variables to represent the three group of workers yielded the same results.

Only for financial hardship and depression is there significant impact of reemployment. Workers who are reemployed have almost equal mean levels of financial hardship and depression as workers who were employed at both waves. Both groups have significantly less financial hardship and depression than workers unemployed at both waves. Therefore, there are demonstrable effects of regaining employment. One is obvious: when one is re–employed, one suffers less financial hardship. The other is somewhat less obvious, but still critical: reemployment lessens depression.

Initial Resources.   As Chapter Two noted, the world did not randomly sort workers into closing and nonclosing plants. In the months before the plants closed, the higher seniority workers had a chance to transfer to (or be recalled to) other plants; thus, workers in closing plants more often had low seniority at GM. Because unskilled workers, the young, women, and racial minorities had lower seniority, they were overrepresented in plants scheduled to close. So were unmarried workers, because they tended to be younger. Over and above the seniority difference, our analyses also indicated that females and minorities were a bit more

Table 3.11

Effects of Reemployment for Closing Plant Workers[a]

	Unemployed Wave 2 Reemployed Wave 3	Unemployed at both Wave 2 and 3	Employed at both Wave 2 and 3
Financial hardship Wave 3	44.70	55.34	46.67[b]
Depression Wave 3	1.47	1.61	1.49[b]
Anxiety Wave 3	1.30	1.45	1.35
Child conflict Wave 3	6.00	6.33	6.09
Spouse conflict	6.66	6.71	6.98

[a] All means are adjusted for covariates: age, sex, education, income, seniority, having a confidant or not, and the wave 1 measure of the dependent variable.
[b] Means differ significantly at p < .05.

likely to remain in closing plants. Only for educational attainment was there no real difference between the workforces of the plants, as of the first wave of the panel study.

The financial hardships that workers experience in the face of an event like a plant closing are, in part, a function of the resources they have available to cushion or buffer the blow of unemployment. Five kinds of financial resources are considered here: the person's own income during the previous year; the person's total family income; family savings; home ownership; and having a spouse who works. We suspected that certain groups which were more likely to be closing plant workers might start out with fewer financial resources. In fact, women always had significantly fewer resources than men, less personal income, less family income, less money saved, and less home ownership. Ironically, they were even slightly less likely to have working spouses, because fewer female workers were married than were males. Blacks were similarly disadvantaged relative to whites, and again in all three survey years. To be young or low in seniority was also linked to having less personal income, less family income, less money saved, less home ownership, and fewer working spouses). Young workers, who are more likely to be unmarried, may suffer an additional, subtle financial deprivation: the lack of the second income a spouse provides. In sum, if low seniority, unskilled, young, female, or minority workers already make less—already feel some financial pinch—a plant closing becomes another case of "the poor get poorer."

Race, Gender, and Jobs

Because some groups such as women and blacks were overrepresented in closing plants, the question arises, Exactly what did happen to their jobs?

Table 3.12 shows the percentage of males versus females, by race, who reported not working either zero, one, two, or three times across the panel study. As Chapter Two noted, we always compare black and white workers, excluding "others" (18 cases as of Wave 1 and 12 cases as of Wave 3), to clarify the meaning of any race effects.

The table shows that both blacks and women were disadvantaged, in comparison to whites and men, but women were the more disadvantaged group. This conclusion emerges most clearly when we asked about steady employment. Over two–thirds of male workers were employed at all three surveys; this was true of less than one–third of women. The difference between white and black men was a more subtle 73% versus 68%. To see where the lower rates of employment for blacks and women came from, first we looked separately at closing versus nonclosing plants. There was no significant difference between blacks and whites in the number of times employed within the nonclosing plants; differences were restricted to the closing plants. The gender difference—women were always more likely to report not being employed, regardless of type of plant—was true regardless

Table 3.12
Autoworkers' Unemployment In the Aftermath of Plant Closings
by Race and Gender [a]

	White		Black	
	Male	Female	Male	Female
N =	705	111	148	83
A. Patterns of unemployment Number of times unemployed across waves[b]				
None	73.0%	32.4%	67.6%	39.8%
One	15.5	36.9	20.9	25.3
Two	10.4	24.3	9.5	22.9
Three	1.1	6.3	2.0	12.0
Mean weeks unemployed/ Looking for work[c]	12.9	24.4	15.7	26.3
B. Patterns of Employment at Wave 3[d] Closing Plants				
Work at GM	10.5%	3.7%	8.8%.	6.2%
Work elsewhere	21.1	38.5	29.3	33.3
Unemployed	10.7	28.4	10.2	25.9
Nonclosing plants				
Work at GM	52.0	16.5	48.3	27.2
Work elsewhere	4.1	10.1	2.0	3.7
Unemployed	1.6	2.8	1.4	3.7
Wave 3 hourly wage:[e]	$15.00	$10.44	$13.89	$11.41

[a] N (1,047) was restricted to workers who had data for all three waves, were not retired by Wave 2 or 3, and were white or black. The question regarding weeks of unemployment was not asked of those who declared themselves out of the labor market temporarily or permanently (hence, N = 937).
[b] Chi–square for cumulative unemployment significant for race ($X^2 = 14.6$, df = 3, p = .002) and for gender ($X^2 = 107.8$, df = 3, p < .0001). Race–gender interaction, ns. In a 2 x 2 ANOVA treating number of times unemployed as continuous, only gender was significant ($F(1,1043) = 90.6$, p < .0001).
[c] In a 2 x 2 ANOVA, the effect of gender was highly significant ($F(1,1043) = 19.8$, p < .0001); neither race nor the race by gender interaction approached significance.
[d] The effect of gender was highly significant within and across race (chi–square = 16.5 among blacks, 72.4 among whites, and 86.8 overall, (df = 5, p < .0001). The effect of race was marginally significant (p = .099) across gender and insignificant within gender (chi–squares of 5.7 among males, 6.3 among females, and 9.2 overall, again with df = 5).
[e] A 2 x 2 ANOVA shows significant effects of gender ($F(1, 838) = 100.73$, p < .0001) and of the gender–race interaction ($F(1, 838) = 8.84$, p = .003).

of the type of plant. Next, we looked at employment for each wave of the survey separately. The lower employment among the closing plant black men compared to white men when they were first interviewed, disappeared by Wave 3. Women, in contrast, were still reporting being unemployed at a higher rate than men, as of Waves 2 and 3.

To sum up, in the wake of the 1987 GM plant closings, both blacks and women were losing their places at GM. But by the end of the study, when we looked at who was employed at GM, blacks were present in almost the same proportions as they had been at the beginning. In contrast, women worked in GM plants only half as often as they once had; they constituted 9% rather than their previous 18% of workers. Literally, those GM plants that remained in operation became more of a "man's world."

Race and Gender Combined

One important remaining issue is whether the combination of race and gender is special in any way. For example, do black females fare particularly poorly? The answer, in a word, is no. Table 3.12 summarizes employment information for the four race–gender combinations. No statistically significant interactions emerged for the effects of race and gender for the number of times a worker was unemployed, the duration of unemployment in weeks, or the nature of employment, as of Wave 3. Race differences were slight and generally insignificant across all of these measures, but gender effects were large. Females experienced more instances of unemployment, had longer lasting unemployment, and (if they were working) were more likely to find themselves at Wave 3 in new jobs rather than working at generally more lucrative GM jobs.

The only evidence of any significant race–gender interaction emerged for hourly wages as of Wave 3. Among men, whites outearned blacks, but the reverse was true for women. Table 3.12 suggests an explanation of this trend: where the women worked. If they were working, black women were more often still at GM, and hence made more money; this earning difference held even when we carried out regressions that controlled for seniority (not shown). At the same time, black women were also more often unemployed than their white counterparts. Overall, the most striking result for either the nature of employment or the pay rate is that for both races, men were more likely than women to work at GM and to make high hourly wages. By the third wave of this panel study, the story of jobs lost and poorer jobs regained was a story of gender, not of race. We saw no evidence that race and gender together produced any sort of interactive "double whammy."

Workers' Other Characteristics

Numerous other differences in personal characteristics existed between workers in closing and nonclosing plants (see Chapter 2).

Table 3.13 shows how other characteristics of workers were related to the frequency of employment. First, predictably, the patterns for seniority and age go hand in hand. Of course, it is the highest seniority workers who are least likely to ever report being out of work. But the next highest seniority is found in a somewhat surprising place: those out of work twice. Two very different forces probably contributed to this trend. First, it is generally found that younger workers are reemployed more rapidly in an event like a plant closing because other employers see them as easier to retrain or cheaper to employ (e.g., Herz, 1991). Second, higher seniority GM workers may have been willing to "wait it out," because they thought their chances of getting back into GM were good. Such workers have repeated experiences with layoffs in the industry, repeated learning experiences that high seniority eventually pays off in the end with a return to the line. We also found that unmarried workers were overrepresented in each category of unemployment. Table 3.13 omits patterns for marital status because these mainly reflect the worker's age. The worker's income at the start of the study, which is itself linked to both seniority and skill level, is linearly related to employment trends. Workers who originally made the most were also the least likely to be without work at any point. Finally, having more education at the outset both protected workers against job loss and helped with reentry into jobs. The stably employed and those who reported being unemployed once had essentially the same educational level, higher than that of the other two groups.

CONCLUSIONS

This chapter has considered the link between expectations and reality. What did the workers expect after the plant closing, and what happened? The simplest answer is that they expected less and they got what they expected. Most thought it would be difficult or impossible to get a job with as good pay and benefits as the GM job, and they were correct. The new jobs that they got came with about one–third less pay and benefits that were significantly inferior to those they had at GM. Some expected that retraining would be required, and it was, particularly for the higher paying jobs.

Our expectations about the characteristics of workers and old and new jobs were also fulfilled. We expected that the older, white, and male workers would

Table 3.13
Characteristics of Workers By Employment Status
(Closing and Nonclosing Plants Combined)[a]

Worker was	Never without job	Without job once	Without job twice	Without job all waves
Seniority at GM (years)	17.9	10.6	16.6	9.4
Age (years)	43.4	37.9	43.2	39.2
Own income in previous year (thousands)	43.1	38.5	38.3	35.7
Education (years)	12.4	12.3	11.7	11.9

[a] Data were obtained in Wave 1. The difference among the four employment categories was highly significant for all variables (p < .0001) by appropriate tests (chi–square or analysis of variance).

begin with more resources and would be more likely to keep their jobs. This expectation was borne out. Closing plant workers were disproportionately young, black, and female. The women in closing plants were particularly hard hit, less likely to find jobs, less likely in be married in the first place, and thus to have the second income a spouse can provide. This is our first look at how hard times differently impact already vulnerable people. Unfortunately, this is a pattern that is repeated in later chapters as well.

4

Feelings: Downsizing's Effects on Individuals and Families

Sometimes all I could do was think about what they had done to me. I felt worthless, but mostly I felt it was GM's fault. But there was no GM to bitch out or get even with. When I couldn't get by any more and I couldn't find a job and I couldn't stand to see anybody I used to work with, I guess I just turned it all on myself. Yeah, I was crazy.
—a closing plant worker

The 1987 GM plant closings were a major upheaval for thousands of workers, for the union that represented those workers, and for the communities they called home. At first, workers recognized that they were bit players in a tragedy not of their own making. As the worker quoted above put it, ". . . mostly I felt it was GM's fault." But workers were shadow boxing with an enemy they could not find, an enemy with whom a fair fight was impossible.

This chapter first assesses the emotional toll that the closing of the plants and/or the unemployment it generated may have caused individual workers. Here we are concerned with symptoms of emotional distress, that is, mild to severe versions of the symptoms that characterize depression, anxiety, and other disorders. We ask whether this distress was concentrated within workers whose plants closed, or also affected workers whose plants stayed open. The second broad theme of the chapter is the effects of plant closing, unemployment, or the financial hardship that accompanies unemployment on the emotional climate of family life. The two main indicators are a) at the extreme, workers' reports of "split–ups"—broken off relationships, separations, or divorces; and, b) in milder form, workers' reports of the frequency of various forms of stress and conflict with spouse or partner and with children. Although the latter may lead to the former, it cannot be assumed that the relationship is automatic.

As Chapter One outlined, the research literature suggests that a basic assumption should be the interconnectedness of moods and feelings in a family. Mental distress in the individual has consequences for the "mental health" of the family and particularly for the behaviors and moods of the spouse or partner. This relationship has been shown most clearly in the case of depression. Put bluntly, depressed people are hard to live with. Their behavior seems to generate distress and eventually rejection from those who live with and care about them. And even though the depressed person may have "started it," the rejection they experience makes their situation worse. Whatever they had to be depressed about, now they have more.

Therefore, our investigation of the feelings of individuals and families closes with a brief investigation of whether these plant closings or the unemployment that accompanied them actually generated a spiral of interconnected distress—individual to family to individual.

DISTRESS OVER TIME

To parallel the employment data reported for the closing versus nonclosing plants, first we provide an overview of depression, anxiety, and somatic symptoms by type of plant across the three waves of the study. This analysis reveals an important finding: Being in a plant that did not close had its stressful side, and we can show it.

Figure 4.1 shows the trends over time for closing and nonclosing plant workers, with separate lines for depression, anxiety, and somatic symptoms. We need to think of these trends in terms of differences between these two groups of workers, differences between types of symptoms, and changes over time. The first thing to expect, of course, is that more evidence of misery — more symptoms of more complaints — is likely to be found in the closing plants. This is generally what the figure shows. The solid lines that stand for the closing plant workers float above the dashed lines that stand for the nonclosing plant workers—not always by much, and not every time, but most of the time, showing a higher misery index in the closing plants. One difference involved the type of symptom. Closing and nonclosing plant workers didn't differ in somatic symptoms, but closing plant workers were always more depressed and anxious than workers whose plants did not close. In terms of their medical importance and economic cost, depression and anxiety are the "big guns" of these three. Closing plant workers suffered most in the ways that hurt the most.

Figure 4.1 also says something about the hidden costs of plant closings over time. We warned early on that this study might underestimate the social and psychological cost of plant closings because our "control" group of nonclosing plant workers, who served as the benchmark against which closing plant workers were always being compared, was also suffering. Figure 4.1 shows ways in which this was true. The trends over time for nonclosing plant workers tell us some important things about being the "control" group in a real–life, highly threatening social change. These workers whose plants didn't close were not immune to the impact of plant closing, any more than closing plant workers were. Looking at their scores in the second and third wave and then looking back at Wave 1, we can see that the anxiety and somatic symptoms — but not depression symptoms — of the nonclosing plant workers were highest at Wave 1. Both of these scores dropped significantly from Wave 1 to Wave 2 and again from Wave 2 to Wave 3 for this group.

It appears that the nonclosing plant workers were almost literally "sweating it out." At first, they were probably not sure that their own plants would remain open. They were afraid of what might happen and what might befall them next week, month, or year. Gradually they relaxed. Their headaches went away. By Wave 3, "no sweat." Closing plant workers also found some relief over time, but less quickly. Their somatic complaints leveled off after Wave 1. Both anxiety and depression dropped after Wave 2.

Comparing the three kinds of distress, it is apparent that closing plant workers were always more depressed than workers whose plants did not close— and this form of distress was relatively resistant to change.

One reason why despair may stick in this way, of course, is something on which social science and common sense have long agreed: Once a person is depressed, it can lead to unemployment, just as surely as unemployment leads to depression. However, because people are not assigned randomly to lose jobs or to keep them, we cannot be completely certain about cause and effect. But a plant closing, in which people lose jobs through no evident fault of their own, offers a chance to explore how depression may contribute to joblessness over time.

Instead of comparing closing with nonclosing plant workers, it is possible to explore trends over time in terms of employment status and its changes by focusing on two waves at a time (in an analysis of variance framework, assessing Employment Status W1 by Employment Status W2, for example). In fact, the same conclusions about overall trends in distress and differences among forms of distress emerge, as Table 4.1 indicates.

The consistently employed have the lowest levels of depression, anxiety, and somatic complaints, whereas the consistently unemployed have generally the highest levels of emotional distress. Although this may be true generally, what is most striking is that employment is far superior to unemployment for mental health. In almost every case, the employed have better mental health than the people who are unemployed. The next set of analyses addresses the fact that eventually it is

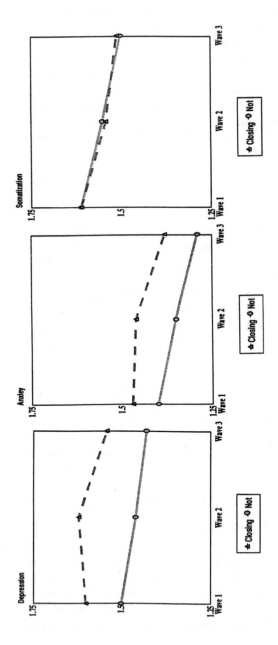

Figure 4.1. Mental health in closing versus nonclosing plants at three points.

Table 4.1

Adjusted Means for Depression, Anxiety, and Somatic Symptoms by
Employment Status Over Time: Repeated Measures Analysis of Covariance[a]

Wave 1 – Wave 2

		Wave 1			
		Employed Wave 2		Unemployed Wave 2	
		Employed	Unemployed	Employed	Unemployed
	N =	674	223	63	47
Wave 1					
Depression		1.49	1.60	1.68	1.75
Anxiety		1.39	1.45	1.57	1.66
Somatic		1.57	1.66	1.61	1.71
Wave 2 Depression		1.45	1.68	1.64	1.73
Anxiety		1.35	1.54	1.43	1.50
Somatic		1.52	1.62	1.54	1.54

Wave 2 – Wave 3

		Wave 2			
		Employed Wave 3		Unemployed Wave 3	
		Employed	Unemployed	Employed	Unemployed
	N =	708	29	133	137
Wave 2					
Depression		1.46	1.61	1.61	1.77
Anxiety		1.35	1.46	1.46	1.60
Somatic		1.52	1.68	1.49	1.71
Wave 3 Depression		1.44	1.64	1.45	1.67
Anxiety		1.31	1.38	1.29	1.46
Somatic		1.48	1.66	1.44	1.63

[a] N = 1,007 workers who had all demographic data and were not retired by Wave 2 or Wave 3. All means are adjusted for effects of seniority at GM, race, gender, marital status, education, age, and worker's income before Wave 1.

employment, rather than closing or nonclosing plant status, that is the decisive determinant of distress.

DEPRESSION AND UNEMPLOYMENT OVER TIME

Are unemployment and poor mental health locked in an unhappy dance of cause and effect, such that poor mental health leads to unemployment, just as unemployment harms mental health? In general, unemployment appears to be linked to a significant but temporary increase in a number of symptoms. Reemployment, the passage of time, or both, lead to a drop in symptoms, often back to baseline levels. Somewhat surprisingly, there is no clear evidence in the previous literature that the distress that follows unemployment leads workers to be any less likely to get reemployed. In fact, one study of the blue–collar unemployed (Kessler, Turner, & House, 1989) found that those who were more anxious or depressed were somewhat more likely, rather than less likely, to become reemployed in the course of a year. The authors pointed out that their results may be specific to the kind of job market these workers were facing, which was an improving market with readily available jobs (see Liem & Liem, 1988). There are important similarities between their study and ours. Kessler et al. (1989) surveyed blue–collar workers (mainly from the auto industry) in southeastern Michigan. Our sample is larger, drawn from the same area a few years later, and is exclusively from auto plants. However, the job market during our data gathering was poorer, and in itself, the scope of the plant closings generated considerable concern that a major downturn would result.

To see whether this was what happened in these plant closings, we concentrate on depression because it was the longest lasting form of distress and the one most closely linked to being in a closing plant. The question becomes, Does depression worsen the worker's situation by helping to keep the worker unemployed? For example, depression could lead the worker to become discouraged—to stop looking or to look less efficiently or enthusiastically.

Independent Variables: Employment Status. First it is important to define the terms, for this chapter begins to look at unemployment through a more restrictive lens or definition. In the analysis of mental health, unemployed refers to all workers who were not employed and not retired at each wave of the survey, whether or not they considered that they were looking for work. We leave the retirees out in these analyses because their mental health was basically the same as that of workers still employed at GM (Even when we leave them in, contrasting the employed and the unemployed, the overall patterns remain the same.) The category employed includes the small number of part–time, as well as the full–time workers.

The Model

Next, we build a model of what reality would look like if unemployment and depression do cause each other and test to see if this model is consistent with the facts. It is important to keep in mind that this model may not be the only explanation of those facts. But if the findings are consistent with a claim that depression leads to unemployment, we will have identified one kind of "double whammy" that can follow from plant closings. If losing a job makes you depressed and being depressed itself makes you less likely to get or to have a job, then a plant closing will lead to some people being hit simply because they are already down.

Figure 4.2 depicts a model of this process. It is a simplified version of the possible predictors in at least two respects. First, it would be possible to trace out a more complex pattern among the initial causes, whereby personal characteristics create seniority which causes a worker to be in a closing or nonclosing plant and causes the worker to be employed or unemployed at Wave 1. However, this would complicate the estimations with little gain in answering the key question here: Does depression lead to as well as follow from unemployment? Second, because of the multicollinearity of the interactions among the personal characteristics and unemployment, it is necessary to sacrifice some of the complexity in the known causes of initial depression (see Hamilton, Broman, Hoffman, & Renner, 1990) to model its relationship to unemployment over time. Figure 4.2 indicates that workers' personal characteristics (the six social statuses in which we are interested), their seniority at GM, and their Wave 1 employment status affect initial levels of depression. At each wave of the survey, the figure shows unemployment leading to depression but not the reverse. Across waves of the survey, both unemployment and depression appear as causes of unemployment in the next wave. (Because depression at any wave of the survey was measured during the interview, whereas the worker's employment status existed before the interview, we do not consider depression a cause of unemployment in the same wave of data.)

We estimate the model using structural equations. In general, the use of a structural model is acknowledged to be superior to the use of cross–correlation to analyze panel data (Kessler & Greenberg, 1981; Rodgers, 1989). An ordinary least squares (OLS) solution for the model has certain advantages. It is readily understood, and its familiar R^2 and increments in R^2 provide indicators of the variance explained in endogenous variables and the relative impacts of predictors. However, when the errors may be correlated across equations, the method of seemingly unrelated regressions (SURE) is more appropriate (Judge, Griffiths, Hill, Lutke, & Lee, 1985). Even using SURE, it could be argued that regressors in the equations for unemployment and depression at Waves 2 and 3 may be correlated with those equations' error terms because of the combination of correlated errors over time and lagged values of unemployment and depression in these equations. However, we are treating these lagged variables as exogenous to the current time period in each equation. In other words, their status is no different from that of other variables such as gender or race. This eliminates the problem of correlations between regressors and error terms. Such a solution is not entirely satisfactory, but with only three time periods it is virtually impossible to employ the common generalized least squares correction for serial correlation. Furthermore, the SURE technique that we employ is a form of generalized least squares which, by correcting for correlated errors across equations for different waves, acts as a correction for serial correlation across waves. Although we estimated the model of Figure 4.2 using both OLS and SURE, an OLS solution is presented in Table 4.2 because of its familiarity to social science readers.

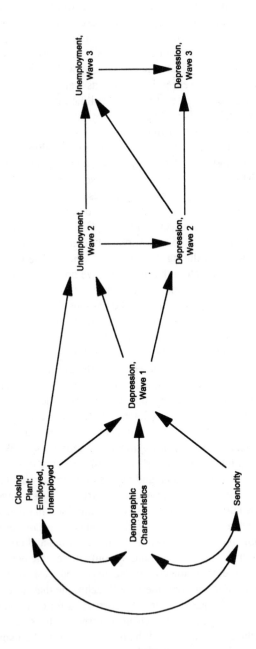

Figure 4.2. Unemployment and depression: linkages over time.

Table 4.2
The Depression–Unemployment Relationship Over Time (OLS Solution)[a]

Wave 1 Depression

Regressor	Unstandardized Coefficient	t–ratio
Intercept	1.95	9.50[c]
Seniority (years)	.01	3.01[c]
Closing (Employed 1)	.04	.43
Closing (Unemployed 1)	.17	2.35[b]
Minority	−.14	−2.90[c]
Female	.33	6.11[c]
Married	−.06	−1.18
Education (years)	−.01	−.44
Age (years)	−.01	−3.19[c]
Prior income (thousands)	−.01	−2.00[b]
$R^2 = .07$		

Wave 2 Unemployment

Regressor	Unstandardized Coefficient	t–ratio
Intercept	−.05	−1.32
Closing (employed 1)	.41	15.56[c]
Closing (unemployed 1)	.33	8.09[c]
Depression 1	.08	4.03[c]
$R^2 = .22$		

Wave 2 depression

Regressor	Unstandardized coefficient	t–ratio
Intercept	.69	15.87[c]
Depression 1	.51	19.53[c]
Unemployment 2	.19	5.22[c]
$R^2 = .31$		

Wave 3 Unemployment

Regressor	Unstandardized Coefficient	t–ratio
Intercept	−.04	−1.54
Unemployment 2	.45	20.27[c]
Depression 2	.05	3.41[c]
$R^2 = .32$		

Wave 3 depression

Regressor	Unstandardized Coefficient	t–ratio
Intercept	.70	17.84[c]
Depression 2	.50	20.72[c]

Unemployment 3	.13	3.20^{c}
$R^2 = .33$		

[a] N = 1,007 respondents.
[b] p < .05.
[c] p < .01.

The results of our analysis are consistent with the figure. For example, how did a worker become unemployed at Wave 2? In three ways: (1) by being unemployed at Wave 1, (2) by being in a closing plant and not yet unemployed at Wave 1, and (3) by being depressed at Wave 1. This was the last evidence of an effect of being in a closing plant, in itself, independent of being unemployed. The distinction between closing and nonclosing plants loses its usefulness, except purely descriptively, as the worker moves through the years of the surveys, that is, it eventually becomes unnecessary to keep track of the origin (closing versus nonclosing plant). The long–term damage of being in a closing plant is "carried"—its mental health meaning is conveyed—by what it does to employment patterns.

Workers became unemployed at Wave 3 in two ways: (1) by being unemployed at Wave 2 and (2) by being depressed at Wave 2. In turn, workers were always more depressed if they had been depressed before and if they were jobless now. These findings are consistent with the argument that there is a two–way street of cause and effect here, one in which unemployment builds depression and depression generates or maintains unemployment. Although it is necessary to be cautious in our interpretation, the data suggest a strong link between the depression and unemployment.

So Were They Crazy?

Thus far this chapter has concentrated on the ways in which the distress of autoworkers manifested itself, grew, or receded. We have not emphasized one very important thing about this distress, one way in which our findings mirror those of earlier studies of plant closings. In some absolute sense, these workers did not report being in extreme distress. Some may have said they were "crazy," as did the worker quoted earlier, but on the whole their reports of symptoms did not indicate that they felt very crazy very often. Then what does it mean for the depression and anxiety and "sweating it out" to have been mild rather than severe, and why was it not worse?

Remember that when we asked about each symptom, workers had five options to describe life in the past 30 days. If they said they didn't have the symptom at all, we scored this a 1. "Some of the time" was scored a 2, "fairly often" a 3, "very often" a 4, and "a great deal" a 5. Instead of noticing the differences between closing and nonclosing plants or the trends over time, one thing we could have emphasized about the distress of these workers is that, on average, they did not say they had any type of symptom as often as "some of the time." (Their average scores were below 2.) One message of these numbers is that these workers were not "disturbed" or suffering from "disorders." They were, if anything, "distressed" about their lives. The numbers should reinforce our early warning that what is at issue here is people who are more or less stressed and distressed by a trying life experience are not people who are or should be hospital patients. They may feel crazy, but clearly there is little evidence of clinically significant symptoms.

One reason why workers did not report more symptoms, or any more frequent symptoms, is that they did not have them. A second reason is the fact that these are things to which people in general don't want to admit and blue–collar workers might find it especially hard to express. What do we expect a group of autoworkers, mostly male, average age over 40, to say when we ask them whether they have been "crying easily" (a symptom of depression)? Even if they have been, will they say so? Perhaps these workers shaded the truth in the direction of looking better to themselves and to the interviewer.

Although this might be true, let us assume for the sake of argument that workers were accurately reporting what they felt. They really were not that bad off. Why not? One reason may lie in what these answers say about people's abilities to get through the day. Consider what it would mean to say "some of the time" in response to each symptom of depression, for example. In their exact wording and in the order they were asked about, these are the 12 symptoms:

loss of sexual interest or pleasure
trouble getting to sleep or staying asleep
thoughts of ending your life
poor appetite
crying easily
a feeling of being trapped or caught
blaming yourself for things
feeling lonely
feeling blue
worrying or stewing about things
feeling no interest in things
feeling hopeless about the future

A way to understand workers' scores is to realize that if a person actually had each of these thoughts and feelings "some of the time" in the past month, it would be a very bad month indeed. A person who was burdened by all of them "a great deal" of the time would have had a hard time making it through our interview. It is consistent with this interpretation of the numbers that an average score of about a "3" on the 1–5 scale is reached among psychiatric inpatients. In a sense, the middle of the scale is the end of the road—where these symptoms reach a level of clinical significance and portend a lack of functioning.

Considering this, it is important not to be complacent about the low numbers here. It is surely true that some of these workers felt anguish. They felt despair. These feelings were real. Still more of the workers felt discomfort, unhappiness, distress — significantly more of it than if a plant had not closed in their lives — but they were still functioning, still getting by.

EFFECTS ON THE FAMILY

> *I was out almost two years and I wanted to get called back.*
> *My wife and I had some trouble, but finally we decided that*
> *she would be the one who went to work. She got in at a*
> *small manufacturing company. We reversed roles—I became*
> *the housewife. Logically it worked out right; it was the*
> *thing to do, but this switching roles brought on a lot of*
> *tension in the house. I was relieved when I got called back*
> *in—we were not doing very well at all for a while.*
> —a closing plant worker

Having a job can be a benefit to workers in at least two ways. It gives us money and therefore dignity in a society where money counts. And it gives us an identity, a role as a worker, and therefore dignity in a society where one's worth is measured by one's work. In a family, the loss of money with loss of work is usually felt by all members of the family. Researchers have realized since the 1930s that unemployment can take a toll on family life. As the classic 1933 study *Marienthal* by Jahoda, Lazarsfeld, & Zeisel (1933) pointed out, good marriages may be strained and bad marriages crushed by the burdens of worry, depression, and fear that settle on households at such a time. And children can carry a legacy of uncertainty and disturbance even into their adult lives (Elder, 1974).

In this section of the chapter, we explore the link between plant closing (and its associated unemployment) and the emotional climate of family life. Several studies have explored this topic, and we provide a review of these studies elsewhere (For a review, see Broman, Hamilton, & Hoffman, 1990). Two issues are explored here. First, were any important ties with spouses or lovers broken as a result of the plant closings? Second, was there more family conflict, either with spouses or children, among workers whose plants closed or who became unemployed?

Broken Ties

As part of the questions on negative life events, we asked workers whether they had experienced breaking off an engagement or affair, separation from a spouse, or divorce. Taken individually, each of these was a rare event at any particular time—involving less than 5% of the workers. Because we know (as shown earlier) that closing plant workers were younger and more often unmarried, it is not surprising that the breaking off of engagements or affairs was always more common in the closing plants than in plants that did not close. Newer marriages are also more fragile, so again it is not surprising that separations were always more common in closing plants. Finally, divorces were somewhat more likely in closing plants by Wave 2 and significantly more likely by Wave 3. What is important is whether there is any trend over time, a trend that might be linked to the plant closings.

Figures 4.3 and 4.4 show the pattern of breakups, separations, and divorces reported in each survey, first for the closing plant workers (Figure 4.3) and then for those whose plants did not close (Figure 4.4). One thing is not surprising about these results. Comparing the two figures, there were clear differences at the outset between closing and nonclosing plant workers. As expected, more broken ties of all sorts occurred in the closing plants.

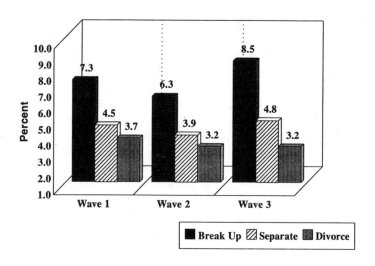

Figure 4.3. Splitting up: broken engagements, separations, and divorces in closing plants.

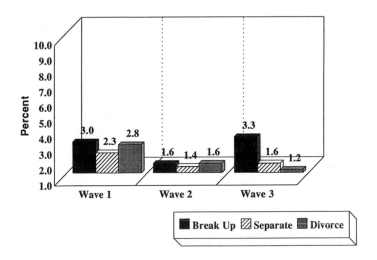

Figure 4.4. Splitting up: broken engagements, separations, and divorces in nonclosing plants.

What is surprising is the trends over time. We had expected that the strain of plant closing might lead more of the closing plant workers to break ties with loved ones as the stress mounted. Instead, the figures show that there is a drop in broken ties at Wave 2 for both closing and nonclosing plant workers. Statistically, this drop is significant in the case of breaking off engagements or affairs, but only for nonclosing plant workers. This serves as a useful reminder to be careful in thinking about linkages between one factor and another. Because social scientists are so used to thinking that a plant closing and job loss make things *worse*, it is important to remember that plant staying open and job keeping can make things *better*. Where broken ties are concerned, any relationship between plant closing and broken ties can reflect the fact that people whose plants close are splitting up more, or that people whose plants don't close are splitting up less, or both. By Wave 3 we see slight increases in the numbers, and the only significant trend involves breaking off engagements or affairs and only among nonclosing plant workers.

Why should this be? First, why would people stay together at higher rates in such times of troubles? There can be many motives for something as complex as not taking action to leave a love relationship. On the positive side, people cling to a loved one for support when troubles come; on the negative side, people who have lost a paycheck may try to stay together with a second person who still has one.

Second, why should this trend appear among workers whose plants do not close? One dictum of social psychology is that happiness and unhappiness are relative. People compare themselves with others to see how they are doing. In the first year or so of our study, the dominant emotion among people whose plants stayed open might have been relief or gratitude for what they had (including loved ones). After all, their lives had just become the greener grass on the other side of a closing plant worker's fence. Alternatively, of course, workers in plants that stayed open may have felt something more like fear or apprehension than gratitude. Uncertainty about the future can make people reluctant to rock the boat in the present.

The workers' answers about family conflict can offer some clues about what underlies the decline in broken ties at Wave 2. For example, if their grass was indeed looking greener, workers in nonclosing plants should report less family conflict over time, or at least no increase in conflict. But if they were clinging to what they saw as flawed relationships because of fear of future economic disaster, conflict could increase.

Causes of Broken Ties. To identify the causes of broken ties, we examine a summary measure for the occurrence of broken ties of any sort. This is a dichotomous measure, which is coded "1" for any broken tie and "0" for those workers who did not report a broken tie.

Table 4.3 shows the contribution of workers' personal characteristics and their job status to the breakup of relationships, concentrating on the third wave of the surveys so we can also look at the cumulative impact of joblessness. Not surprisingly, older workers and those who were married at Wave 1 were significantly less likely to report breaking a tie. We used our measure of marital status as of Wave 1 and broken ties as of Wave 3 to avoid the near tautology (i.e., marriage at any given wave is highly negatively correlated with divorce at that wave). Three other factors which require comment were significant. First, being a minority is associated with breaking family related ties. Financial hardship also has this positive relationship with breaking ties. Minorities and those who experience financial hardship are at an increased likelihood of breaking family ties. On the other hand, having a child living in the household decreases the likelihood of breaking up. This is a pattern which has been found in other research (White, Booth, & Edwards, 1986).

Summary. Broken ties are relatively rare in these data, but they occur more often for those who are young, minority, unmarried, childless, and who suffer financial hardship. We examined the possibility of a statistical interaction between the demographic characteristics and financial hardship. We found no evidence of an interaction of this type. Clearly, some family ties suffer from the stress of the plant closing experience. Another way to think about these numbers is to realize that the illness and death of relationships is a kind of health hazard which is faced more

Table 4.3
Wave 3 Determinants of Broken Ties[a]
Unstandardized Coefficient

Intercept	.29
Seniority (years)	.00
Employed (Wave 3)	−.03
Minority	.05[b]
Female	.02
Married (Wave 1)	−.08[c]
Education	.01
Age	−.01[c]
Prior income	.00
Child in household (Wave 3)	−.06[c]
Financial hardship (Wave 3)	.002[c]
N =	992
R^2 =	.108

[a] N restricted to workers who had data for all three waves.
[b] $p < .05$.
[c] $p < .01$.

often by workers whose plants close. It is faced more often partly because workers whose plants *don't* close try to hang on to what they've got. Next we explore whether they hang on out of gratitude for the known or fear of the unknown.

Family Conflict

In this section, we utilize the measures of family conflict described in Chapter Two. First we report on the specific answers workers gave to each of these questions and on the average level of conflict they reported experiencing with spouse and with children.

How often did workers quarrel with or scream at or even hit their loved ones?

Table 4.4 shows workers' answers to our direct questions about family conflict. The numbers are presented separately for closing, then nonclosing plant workers, for each survey in turn. For simplicity, we compared the most popular response, "never," to all other answers combined. The table shows how many workers said they *ever* did each of the things listed.

First let us get a sense of the general trends and tendencies. It is important to put the answers about "ever" in the context of their reverse—the overwhelming tendency of workers to say they *never* do the things we asked about. For example, even in closing plants, more than one–quarter of workers claimed that they "never" quarrel with their spouse. What are we to make of these findings? Any of the specific numbers here may underestimate the true level of conflict because of

Table 4.4
Frequency of Family Stress Indicators:
Percentage Who Ever Do Each of the Following[a]

	Wave 1 Closing	Non closing	Wave 2 Closing	Non closing	Wave 3 Closing	Non closing
With spouse						
Quarrel	72[b]	55	73[b]	65	79	74
Get on nerves	78[b]	65	73	68	79	75
Scream	43[b]	29	41[b]	28	41	38
Hit	3[b]	1	1	1	1	2
With children						
Arguments	48	42	43	45	53	51
Get on nerves	67[b]	59	61	61	67	64
Lose temper	34	29	26	26	28	26
Hit, slap, or spank	25[b]	17	19	19	26[b]	17

[a] N is restricted to workers who had data at all three waves (range = 837 to 955).
[b] Closing plant workers significantly different from those in nonclosing plants at $p < .05$.

workers' reluctance to report it. Underreporting may be particularly likely for a question like the one about hitting or pushing your spouse. However, there is no reason why underreporting should happen only in plants that close, so we would expect that even though family stress is underreported, the comparison between closing and nonclosing plants is valid. In other words, everyone will underestimate the extent to which they experience family stress.

Are there couples who really never quarrel? We doubt it. But people who say they never quarrel probably don't do so very often. Just as autoworkers have basically good physical health, they appear—by their own reports—to have healthy family lives.

The two rarest forms of conflict, as expected, were hitting of either a spouse or a child. As these workers tell it, almost no one ever pushes or hits a spouse. Similarly, hitting, slapping, or spanking one's child is the least common of the forms of conflict with children (and the second least common overall, behind only "hitting spouse"). Hitting of spouse or child was so infrequent that it was basically unrelated to job loss, to most personal characteristics, or even to the other answers about conflict. (And as we noted earlier, for these reasons, our summary scales for family conflict do not even include the questions about hitting.)

Family Conflict: Group Differences. At Wave 1, Table 4.4 shows a clear difference between workers in closing and nonclosing plants. For every question, closing plant workers reported greater conflict in the family. The superscripts in the table show that this difference was significant in all cases, except for loss of temper with one's child. Over time, however, the difference between the groups fades. Significant differences become less common in Wave 2 and all but disappear in Wave 3.

What does this convergence between workers in closing and nonclosing plants mean? In this case, the convergence occurs because family conflict for closing plant workers tends to stay the same or drop a bit, but the levels of conflict stay the same or rise for workers in the nonclosing plants. This pattern for the closing plant workers is understandable if we imagine that they suffer an initial shock and anger, which gradually wears off (or is replaced by the gratitude for reemployment). But what about workers whose plants did not close? Why would their conflict rise?

It is possible that these trends in nonclosing plants indicate what we have suggested earlier, that some relationships *that would otherwise be broken off* are being held together by fear and uncertainty. The family life of a worker who might otherwise have been leaving—or being left by—a spouse or partner is not likely to be as pretty as the family life of those who really wish to be there. Of course, various other factors may contribute to these findings. But the patterns are at least consistent with the interpretation that fear of the future, rather than satisfaction with the present, led to the decline in broken ties among nonclosing plant workers shown earlier.

Family Conflict Measures

Table 4.5 presents the results of an analysis of differences in family conflict between closing and nonclosing plant workers as measured by our scales. From the table, we see that there are no differences in child conflict between closing and nonclosing plant workers, differences at two of three times in hit, slap, or spank, and differences at all three times in spousal conflict. Where differences are significant, workers in the closing plants report more family conflict. Though the numbers for child conflict are not statistically significant, the trend is still in the direction that

Table 4.5
Differences Between Workers on Measures of Family Conflict

| | Wave 1 status | | |
	Closing	Control	N
Child conflict			
Wave 1	6.14	5.72	779
Wave 2	5.70	5.60	842
Wave 3	6.00	5.77	883
Hit, slap, or spank child			
Wave 1	1.45	1.30[a]	775
Wave 2	1.32	1.32	833
Wave 3	1.45	1.29[a]	877
Spousal conflict			
Wave 1	6.74	5.60[a]	787
Wave 2	6.56	5.72[a]	785
Wave 3	6.84	6.36[a]	792

[a] Differences significant at $p < .05$.

the closing plant workers report more family conflict.

Explaining Family Conflict. Because we already know that workers in closing plants differ demographically from those in nonclosing plants, our analysis of family conflict is incomplete without an examination of the demographic factors in family conflict.

Table 4.6 presents the results of a multiple regression analysis of family conflict measures on demographic variables. We also include negative life events and having a confidant as control variables. Child conflict is predicted by race and sex. The direction of the coefficients indicates that whites and females are more likely than minorities and males, respectively, to report child conflict. The most telling factor leading to family conflict is age. As expected, younger workers said they had more conflict with their spouses and were more likely than older workers to have hit their children. Experiencing negative life events increases family conflict, whereas having a confidant decreases the likelihood of hitting one's child. Not surprisingly, people who have a child living in the household were more likely to report conflict and hitting of children.

In our previous research (Broman et al., 1990) focusing on only Wave 1, we found evidence to suggest a particular pattern of factors that led to family conflict about employment and finances. We found that financial hardship, alone, increased family conflict. We see a similar pattern in these data. Employment status and prior income have no impact on family conflict. Financial hardship, in contrast, is significant. Workers who experience financial hardship also experience more family conflict. Of course, financial hardship was a "family affair," for it included such

Table 4.6
Predictors of Family Conflict

	Child conflict	Hit child	Spousal conflict
Intercept	4.09	2.46	7.39
Seniority (years)	.02	.00	.02
Employed (Wave 3)	.10	−.02	.15
Minority	−.67[b]	.04	−.03
Female	.73[b]	−.05	.18
Education	.30	.02	.16
Age (years)	−.03	−.02[a]	−.05[b]
Prior income (thousands)	.11	.00	−.01
Confidant (1=yes)	.12	−.33[b]	−.53
Negative life events	.16[a]	.02	.34[b]
Child in household (Wave 3)	1.98[b]	.25[b]	−.01
Financial hardship (Wave 3)	.01[a]	.00	.03[b]
N =	846	840	760
R² =	.20	.17	.14

[a] p < .05.
[b] p < .01.

family wide changes as having inadequate food or clothes as well as some changes that specifically touched children—activities on which children might have to cut back (See Chapter Five). We can expect, for example, that a child whose parents can no longer afford summer camp may be less happy as a result. Financial hardship is likely to pervade and poison the emotional climate of the home like few other issues.

As one closing plant worker put it:

After the plant closing, I went to school for computers through the Human Resource Center. My wife went to work, but we have children. So between my schooling and her job, we did what we could to keep the house together. After I graduated from school in computer drafting, I couldn't find a job. Well, I ended up working as a retail clerk in warehousing. I went from $14.00 to $6.80 and now I am at $9.00—the top of my labor grade. This has an effect on things at home. It is stressful. We were young and upgrading our lifestyle and then lost it all. **The family is just not the same. It isn't the home it was.** (Emphasis added).

—a closing plant worker

Workers who suffer from hardship also suffer from—or inflict—conflict with loved ones. The higher the level of hardship experienced, the higher the level of conflict. If job loss brings hardship, and to the extent that job loss brings hardship, these trends tell us that it leads to quarrels and conflict in the home.

A word of caution is in order about interpreting these findings. It is important that we not "write off" these trends because they seem to show that the effects of plant closing on family life are relatively subtle. The upheaval caused by plant closings cannot be entirely captured in such contrasts as closing versus nonclosing, employment versus unemployment, or even in fine–tuned gradations of financial hardship. In part it should be measured in whether workers can even give reasonable answers to the questions. For at least some of the workers, it is more accurate to say that the plant closings made their family life *artificial*, rather than *conflict–filled*. This was likely to happen when workers had to relocate to find work. Afterward, their contact with the family was fundamentally transformed.

As one worker described it:

I was unemployed for a long time and things were getting tougher at home. I got the chance to take a transfer to another facility several states away. I had to take it and leave my family behind in Michigan . . . It is not so easy to be so far from home. But I wouldn't move my family here. I own a house in Michigan, and my kids are in school there. I can't just uproot them and bring them here. I don't know if it would work out. So, every few weeks or so, some of us carpool and head back for two days. I should be there with my family . . . but what can I do? (Emphasis added).

—a closing plant worker

In a case like this, it is not clear how accurate a worker's answers would be about family conflict. If the worker sees no family conflict, this may be only because the worker is not there. When the worker is there, we can be sure that the time together is not "normal" family time. In plant closings, families can be torn apart and family life fundamentally changed *without* any divorce or separation happening. In such cases, questions about "family conflict" do not capture what has happened to spouses, or children, or the workers' ways of touching and being touched by each.

It is worth noting that when we originally conceived of this chapter, we thought we would include a section on negative life events that involved the spouse or a child. Simply put, we found little evidence that events involving family members were linked to unemployment. There was some relationship between financial hardship and financially related events involving family members, but this is to be expected given that the financial hardship experienced by workers is also experienced by their families.

Mental Health and Family Stress

The relationship between the worker's mental health and their family lives is of some interest. There is a clear pattern we can report, but it comes with a clear and important caveat. The pattern is simple; workers who have more distress report more family conflict. This pattern is significant for conflict with the spouse and of borderline significance for conflict with children. The caveat is critical, however. Because workers report on both their mental health and their family conflict, it is possible, perhaps even likely, that the two measures are contaminated by each other. There is no way of being certain if the distress that workers feel causes them to perceive that there is greater conflict in the family, or if there actually is greater conflict. There is also no way of being certain what the correct causal pattern is, from distress to family conflict, or vice versa.

In this sense, we feel we have reached the limits of our analysis with respect to family conflict. Recall that this was not one of our central concerns. Therefore, we did not take pains to measure the constructs from both workers and another family "reporter" (i.e. spouse or children). This is a very difficult task, involving a great deal of time and money, and it is not usually attempted in family studies. Because other concerns were more central for us, we also did not attempt it. Therefore, although we can provide some evidence about a reciprocal relationship between mental health and family conflict, we cannot be definitive. Then, we must leave the reader with our simple finding and its caveat: workers with high distress were more likely to report greater spousal conflict, but because of deficiencies in measurement, the meaning of the pattern is not clear.

CONCLUSIONS

On balance, the most striking finding here was the steady toll that financial hardship takes on family harmony. More subtly, this overview has also suggested a number of ways in which plant closing may damage family life, even among workers whose plants did not close.

When we first encountered them at Wave 1, the workers in closing plants were already in the bleaker future that nonclosing plant workers feared. It showed at home. With regard to splitting up, for example, closing plant workers had about the same levels of divorce, separation, and breakup at the end of our study as at the start. Over time, broken ties and tension and strain with spouse and children generally remained the same or dropped in the closing plants. In contrast, nonclosing plant workers did less breaking up with spouses and lovers around the middle of our study, during the year after the closing of the plants, but their levels of conflict began to rise and stayed high. We suggested that these workers may have been hanging on to what they had, but in fear rather than in gratitude.

What all of these results mean is simple. Work is good for families. Plant closings are bad for families. And plant closings may wreak silent damage, even among those who have not yet reached the end of the line.

5

The Structure of Stress: Workers' Characteristics and the Stress Process

Many stressful experiences, it should be recognized, don't spring out of a vacuum but typically can be traced back to surrounding social structures and people's locations within them. The most encompassing of these structures are the various systems of stratification that cut across societies, such as those based on social and economic class, race and ethnicity, gender, and age. To the extent that these systems embody the unequal distribution of resources, opportunities, and self–regard, a low status within them may itself be a source of stressful life conditions. (Pearlin, 1989:242)

The story of workers' characteristics in this chapter does not begin with a quote from a worker for a simple reason: Closing plant workers did not talk about themselves in this language. Discussions of plant closing or job loss did not lead them to dwell on their gender, race, age, income, education, or (for the most part) their marriages. They talked mostly about unemployment (Chapter Three); later we will turn to the effects of the experience on financial hardships and on the sense of self (Chapter Six). Overall, however, closing plant workers did not reflect upon the way their own characteristics—especially the immutable ones like age or race or gender—might shape their own responses to the stress of plant closing or potential employers' responses to their attempts to regain jobs.

To be more precise, they did not reflect upon these things with us. This is understandable for at least two reasons. First, when they assess why something has happened or what to do about it, people commonly focus upon the situation rather than upon themselves or their own role in it (Jones & Nisbett, 1972). From the worker's viewpoint, discussions of the closings of the plants and the unemployment that followed have a simple focal point: General Motors. In addition to this general tendency of actors to view their situations by looking outward toward other causes rather than inward toward their own roles and identities, it is understandable that workers not focus on characteristics that are essentially immutable for practical reasons (one's sex) or logical reasons (prior income), or that may take substantial effort to alter (educational attainment). Workers tend to talk about not "who I am" but "what I can do" to make things better.

Yet on a theoretical level, the message since Chapter One has been that the worker's identity does matter. Empirically, we have regularly controlled for the effects of various demographic characteristics in analyses, but without considering in detail the kinds of effects of these characteristics might have or their importance. As Chapter One indicated, we conceive of the worker's personal characteristics, which would be considered mostly demographic characteristics, as resources (or liabilities). In the stress process/life course model presented in the figures in Chapter One, workers' personal characteristics and their effects appear as arrow(s).

To have one identity—to be in one demographic category rather than another—can convey economic, social, and cultural capital. When caught in the web of a downsizing event like a plant closing, some workers may be better able than others to "buy their way out" by using these resources.

This chapter will address which characteristics should theoretically matter, as well as why and how they matter in the stress process . It will test whether these workers, under this set of circumstances, fall into line with expectations based on the stress literature. Chapter One also noted that workers' own characteristics serve as resources/liabilities in at least two senses. First, workers who have one or another set of characteristics may be exposed to the stressor to a greater extent; second, such workers may be more reactive or vulnerable to that stressor. We will explore both of these issues.

AT THE BEGINNING OF THE END: WORKERS' REACTIONS AT WAVE 1

Before we can fully consider the issue of stress and mental health among our sample, we must first address some issues of method. The fundamental issue concerns sample attrition and what effect, if any, it might have on the results which we discuss later. Quite simply, if we draw conclusions about responses from Wave 1 based on all the workers who answered at that time, these conclusions might be different from those we would draw if we looked at all workers who responded throughout the surveys. Because of the nature of the modeling we employ in the book, primarily OLS regression, we must select members of the sample who responded to all waves of data collection. Therefore, analyses of change in distress over time or of the influence of unemployment over time restricted the sample based on the answers to three questions:

1. Did the worker provide data about all the predictors of distress we wish to assess (such as demographics, unemployment)?
2. Did the worker respond across all waves of the panel survey (and therefore provide answers about each measure of distress?
3. Was the worker either white or black? (This last restriction served to make the meaning of race effects clear, should those emerge.)

The analyses following are drawn mainly from results for the more inclusive sample (all the Wave 1 responders who fulfill relevant criteria from 1–3 above). Where relevant, we mention ways in which the results are changed by restricting the cases to workers who responded at all waves.

Measures of Distress. This chapter concentrates on the results for depression, the most common mental health consequence of unemployment (Kessler et al., 1988, 1989). For brevity, we omit anxiety, somaticization, and hostility; these measures have a less powerful or long–standing linkage to unemployment in these data. In any case, results for these other measures of distress followed the same patterns as the findings shown here for depression.

In addition to abbreviating the discussion of distress, we have tried to streamline the reporting of results. Results that have been previously published in articles are summarized verbally rather than presented in any detail. The tables and figures are used mainly to convey new information from analyses performed specifically for this book.

Models: Controlling for Selection. The main mechanism for selection into closing versus nonclosing plants and in turn, into unemployment versus continued employment, was seniority at GM. Therefore, given the methodological importance of taking potential selection bias into account, it is important to note that once we took into account workers' personal characteristics as of Wave 1, seniority at GM had no effect on their distress. Therefore, seniority serves as a kind of neutral partner to the other variables in the Wave 1 analyses, and although it was statistically unimportant, it was not deleted because of its methodological centrality to the investigation (e.g., Hamilton et al., 1990).

Models and Variables. As described in Hamilton et al. (1990), in Wave 1 we followed the exploratory tactic of testing for the significance of interactions sequentially, then together, and then trimming away insignificant interactions. An interim model arrived at by that tactic included interactions of race, education, and income with unemployment and of gender with marital status. The final model added a three–way term for race, education, and unemployment to satisfactorily capture the patterns of results. Analyses for this book comparing the Wave 1 full N and for N restricted to those who remained in the panel survey simply reproduced the interim and final models with the differently sized samples.

As of Wave 1, some workers within closing plants were already unemployed, whereas the bulk of workers were anticipating potential unemployment (see Chapter Two). As in Chapter Four's analysis of the depression–unemployment relationship over time, all attempts to predict Wave 1 distress in fact include two terms (unemployed and anticipating unemployment) where only one (unemployed) is needed in later surveys. Therefore, following, we refer to the two terms, although these do not apply to later analyses.

Interim equations for Wave 1 included unemployment (and anticipation), seniority at GM (as a control for selection), age, race, income, education, gender, marital status, the gender–marital status interaction, and the race–unemployment, race–anticipation, income–unemployment, income–anticipation, education–unemployment, and education–anticipation interactions; the final model for each measure of distress added the race–education and race–education–unemployment (and race–education–anticipation) interactions to produce a full test of the three–way relationship among the latter variables. We also refer for simplicity to the effects of "unemployment" when in fact, Wave 1 results represent an amalgam of the effects of unemployment and its anticipation.

Results

General Costs of Workers' Characteristics. Before the plants had even closed, workers' mental health was affected by both their personal characteristics (see Hamilton et al., 1990) and their past experiences (see Calvin, Hamilton, Broman, & Hoffman, 1996 and Chapters Six and Seven of this volume). In each case, the effects were of two major types. First, certain general costs were attached to holding a certain identity or having a certain kind of experience. With regard to personal characteristics, the literature on stress shows that to be female, unmarried, less educated, have low income, and in some cases to be young is to be at a mental health disadvantage (e.g., Kessler et al., 1985; Snyder & Nowak, 1984; Thoits, 1995). Consistent with this literature, in addition to the impact of unemployment itself, we found that at Wave 1 significant mental health costs were attached to being
    female
    unmarried
    young
    less educated
    of lower income
To be in each of these categories or have each of these characteristics was associated with distress, regardless of whether workers were in closing plants or not and regardless of whether or not they still had jobs. These findings tell one story why closing plant workers might be more distressed than workers whose plants don't close: because certain groups of people are more distressed in general, and more of them happen to have suffered through the plant closings.

Complications: The Question of Race. Thus far, we have not mentioned race. It demands more attention, in part because of the nature of this sample. Chapter One noted that "race" differences can be contaminated by class differences in studies of mental health among the general population, that is, differences attributed to race are actually due to differences in the social classes generally occupied by blacks versus whites. Given this, the data set created by our research on the 1987 GM plant closings offer an unusually pure point of comparison. Plant closings in general encompass workers who share a social class but who differ to at least some extent in both the income and the education often used as indicators of class. In fact, the job losses occurred within a single occupation and even a single employer, not only within a single class.

Race can also interact with factors such as class, rather than simply be confounded with them. The most relevant research, by Kessler & Neighbors (1986), tested for interactions between race and class, and the latter was indexed by income and education. These authors reanalyzed data from eight surveys, and modified the statistical models to include race–income and race–education interactions. They found that the impact of income was significantly more pronounced among blacks (or, phrased in terms of race, that race differences in distress were larger among those with lower incomes). Results for education were mixed, and Kessler & Neighbors concluded that '. . . the interaction between race and income is real, whereas the interaction between race and education is either an artifact or a substantive pattern that lacks generalizability to the total U.S. population' (Kessler & Neighbors, 1986, p. 112). Overall, their results suggest that race interacts with at least some indicators of class such that race differences are larger toward the bottom of the stratification pyramid. Therefore we explored the roles of education versus income in interaction with race. Because education is likely to be a more important human capital variable than income from the point of view of reemployment, we expected that education would interact more powerfully with race in this sample. In fact, no significant interaction of race with income emerged at any wave of the panel survey. Therefore, the discussion following concentrates on the way education and race together moderate the impact of unemployment.

Wave 1 : Race. Overall, as of Wave 1, blacks were less distressed than whites (see Hamilton et al., 1990 for these and other results). This finding may have at least two sources. First, it is consistent with the argument that much of the "race" difference often found for mental distress is really a class difference; in other words, take a person's class into account, and the "race" effect vanishes (Kessler et al., 1985). Further, jobs on the line at GM were likely to be seen by blacks as advantageous. Insofar as people evaluate well–being and self–worth relative to similar others and blacks may have assessed their well–being relative to other blacks (Broman, Jackson, & Neighbors, 1989; Rosenberg, 1979), the blacks in this sample should show mental health at least equivalent to their white counterparts.

A significant three–way interaction also emerged among race, education, and unemployment. We expected that as we moved from high education to low education, we also would move from a lower depression score to a higher one (employed, then not employed; high education, then low education). Indeed, this was the pattern we found. In addition, our analyses revealed racial differences in sensitivity to educational levels (black distress levels varied more with education) and differences in sensitivity to unemployment as a function of race and education combined (less educated blacks were severely affected, and more educated blacks were least affected by unemployment).

Other Contingencies. In addition to the effects of workers' characteristics already noted, other contingent relationships emerged between the worker characteristics themselves or between worker identities and unemployment. One such relationship complemented the race–education results just discussed: Income and unemployment interacted such that the impact of unemployment was greater on workers who had lower prior incomes. This can be straightforwardly understood in terms of the financial resources available for dealing with the new source of financial stress.

Gender promised to be an interesting further source of contingent relationships. As Chapter One noted, research on gender differences in response to unemployment has tended to show that males are more sensitive than women to unemployment and other financial losses, but the studies have often failed to look at men and women in the same occupations or financial circumstances; in addition, more recent studies seem to show that this gender gap is disappearing (Caplan et al., 1989). A further frequently studied relationship is the link between gender and marital status in determining distress. The usual finding is that marriage makes a bigger difference in men's mental health than it does in women's, although it is often unclear the extent to which this results from marriage actually helping men or because more mentally healthy men tend to be "selected into" marriage (Forthofer, Kessler, Story, & Gotlib, 1996; Gove, 1972). Finally, speculation about the male "provider" role (see Chapters Six and Seven) suggests that gender, marriage, and employment status may be intertwined determinants of distress. To the extent that a male is satisfying the role of provider (married and employed), he should have the best mental health of all the gender–marriage–employment combinations. At the same time, when a married male loses a job, it represents a threat to an important identity; thus married men who become unemployed should show the largest effect of unemployment on mental health. The calculus of unemployment is not solely financial; an important identity like "provider" can be an asset in one circumstance, a liability in another. Therefore, the effects of gender and employment status, gender and marital status, and their three–way combination appeared likely in this sample of male and female autoworkers.

In fact, as of Wave 1, the only significant contingency involving gender proved to be a gender–marital status interaction. The impact of a worker's marital status on distress depended on gender. Consistent with prior research, married men were much less depressed than their unmarried counterparts, but marital status didn't make a difference in the (high) levels of depression reported by women. It was also true that employment status mattered more to the married men than to anyone else—unemployment generated distress—but the three–way interaction was not significant.

Summary. As of Wave 1, there was limited evidence of differential worker vulnerability to unemployment as a stressor. The three–way interrelationship among race, education, and unemployment shown before is one example of such vulnerability. It can probably most parsimoniously be thought of as involving vulnerability to unemployment based on education, but the impact of education differs for whites and blacks. The fact that the impact of unemployment was greater for those who had a lower initial income was consistent with interpreting unemployment's impact largely in financial hardship terms .

Gender's impact on distress seemed less tied to financial issues like unemployment *per se* and more connected to the identity–conferring roles men and women play. We suggested that the provider role of men might lead to a three–way interaction of gender, marital status, and unemployment (so that the impact of unemployment was greatest for the married men, who had the most to lose in identity terms, as well as in sheer finances). However, both this interaction and the gender–unemployment effect that we predicted were insignificant as of Wave 1. The fact that the only contingency involving gender that emerged was a gender–marital status interaction should be interpreted cautiously. It is important to remember that the Wave 1 surveys occurred *even before the plants had closed.* Unemployment was not yet widespread and it had not become prolonged. Therefore, a fairer test of the role of gender in the response to this stressor required a longer term look at the question of men, women, and their vulnerabilities.

Next Steps

The remainder of the chapter addresses three broad questions:
1. Where did workers stand at the end of two years? What was their distress as of Wave 3, and how was it linked to their personal characteristics?
2. How does this final position stack up relative to workers' initial condition? In other words, does looking at change in distress from Wave 1 to Wave 3 lead to any conclusions different from simply looking at Wave 3 on its own?
3. What role does the accumulation of unemployment play in generating and maintaining of distress? How does the picture look as of Wave 3 if we replace "Wave 3 unemployment" as an independent variable with a familiar measure like number of times unemployed? Does either distress or change in distress seem differently linked to workers' identities when the measure is cumulative rather than a "spot check"?

OVER THE LONG RUN: METHODOLOGY

The third time we talked to these workers, two years had gone by since the closing of the plants. As before, the statistical models take into account six personal characteristics — race, gender, marital status, education, age, and prior income — plus seniority at GM. Because of losses from the sample between surveys (from 1,597 to 1,136), certain categories of worker characteristics or combinations of categories were very small. The bottom line is that multivariate regressions may not provide reliable estimates of effects, especially for complex relationships like the three–way race–education–unemployment interaction.

This difficulty in analyzing complex combinations of characteristics is not new. We have already encountered it both theoretically, in Chapter One, and empirically, in the discussion of Wave 1 results. It is a recurring tension in the sociological study of stress that if and when we really understand all the factors that impinge upon a person and how those factors work, we are talking about biography more than about sociology. Every N is ultimately one. Here we attempt to 'have it both ways' by doing the usual statistical tests but combining these tests with descriptive detail about configurations of worker characteristics like the race–education–unemployment or gender–marital status–unemployment combinations.

Choice of Statistical Approaches

A second set of issues arises in the analysis of panel data such as these: what to focus on as the independent variable and what to focus on as the dependent variables. By questioning the independent variable, we mean to ask about unemployment and to ask whether the key concern is unemployment, as it affects distress at the end of the study (Wave 3 unemployment), versus unemployment, as it has accumulated across the panel study (a measure like the number of times unemployed). In questioning the dependent variables, the issue is not whether to choose depression or anxiety or whatever. The issue concerns whether the focus should be on distress—of whatever sort—as of Wave 3, or on change in distress since Wave 1. Together, these two dimensions of questions generate four strategies for data analysis, each with different implications for the inferences that can be drawn. These are summarized in Figure 5.1.

We actually analyzed the data in all four ways suggested in the figure, although we do not present all of them here. Instead we seek first to understand what can be gained by each way of looking at the issue. It is possible to foresee which of the combinations presented in Figure 5.1 will be the most and least stringent approach to the Wave 3 data. First, the use of Wave 1–Wave 3 change scores should be the most stringent approach because it minimizes certain effects. For example, to the extent that a worker characteristic like gender is a pervasive, continuing determinant

Independent Variable (Unemployment)

Dependent Variable(s) (Distress)	Wave 3 Unemployment	Unemployment Wave 1-Wave 3 (Duration/Extent)
Wave 3 Distress	<u>a</u> Describes Wave 3 distress (no control for prior distress; no assessment of the role of prior unemployment)	<u>b</u> Assesses the impact of extent of prior unemployment on distress as of Wave 3
Change in Distress Wave 1 - Wave 3	<u>c</u> Shows impact of change in distress between Wave 1 and Wave 3	<u>d</u> Shows impact of extent of prior unemployment (and other predictors) on change in distress between Wave 1 and Wave 3

Figure 5.1. Alternative approaches to analysis of wave 3 data.

of distress, gender is not likely to show up as a significant determinant of change in distress over a two–year period. Using change scores can also hide effects related to a changing case base. For example, in analyses of the effects of accumulated unemployment on raw Wave 3 distress, we observed a change in the role of seniority at GM. Seniority was associated with greater distress by Wave 3, rather than being unrelated to distress. Once we observed this new pattern for seniority, we backtracked to the Wave 1 data because we suspected that attrition from the sample was the cause of this change. When Wave 1 data were restricted to those workers who remained in the sample throughout the panel study, the "Wave 3 effect" (where seniority was linked to higher distress) was also produced as of Wave 1. This kind of result with seniority probably reflects the fact that highly distressed workers with high seniority are likely to remain in the sample because they are waiting for work to open up again at GM; low seniority workers, in contrast, leave and are lost from the sample at a higher rate. This exploration of seniority illustrates that the apparent effects of stress can change over time as a function of the shifting groups of people who are interviewed. Such an effect obviously cannot be observed at all by exclusively analyzing change scores, because they eliminate respondents who leave a sample.

Turning to the other dimension of analysis, the independent variable, it is evident that using accumulated unemployment to predict distress adds information over and above that provided by current (Wave 3) unemployment. For example, the worker who is unemployed as of Wave 3 may also have accumulated hardships and scars as a result of one (or two) prior unemployment experiences; the weight of both the current and the accumulated hardship is felt together in the omnibus variable. Therefore a variable like ours that taps the number of times unemployed should logically offer the most chance to observe an effect of unemployment and its potential interactions.

Taking the dimensions of Figure 5.1 together, it was our expectation that the most stringent and restricted view of the data would be provided by using change scores for the dependent variables, as predicted by current (Wave 3) unemployment. The approach that we felt would offer the maximum opportunity to find relationships would be using raw Wave 3 distress scores as the dependent variable in combination with accumulated unemployment as the independent variable. In terms of the lettered boxes in Figure 5.1, the most stringent approach is cell c, whereas the most expansive is cell b. This chapter presents findings from cells a and c together (that is, Wave 3 distress predicted by Wave 3 unemployment; Wave 1–Wave 3 change in distress predicted by Wave 3 unemployment). This combination provides a direct parallel to the original Wave 1 analyses of distress scores, via cell a, and a stringent test of change over time via cell c. Where relevant, as in the discussion of the seniority results in the previous paragraph, the chapter summarizes results from the other analyses. In general, we hope that the figure and the multiple analyses help to illustrate the variety of answers that can be obtained in a panel study as a function of the questions asked and the tools used.

Table 5.1
Impacts of Race, Gender, and Wave 3 Unemployment on
Symptoms of Depression and the W1–W3 Change in Depression
(Standardized Coefficients) [a]

	Model I Baseline	Model II Race	Model III Gender
Unemployed (U)			
Beta (depression)	.14[c]	.58[b]	.17[c]
Beta (change score)	.11[c]	.78[c]	.15[c]
Black (B) Beta (depression)	−.06	−.05	−.06
Beta (change score)	−.02	−.01	−.02
Female (F) Beta (depression)	.14[c]	.14[c]	.17[c]
Beta (change score)	.05	.04	.08[b]
Seniority (S) Beta (depression)	.07	.07	.07
Beta (change score)	.02	.02	.02
Age (A) Beta (depression)	.09[b]	−.09[b]	−.08[b]
Beta (change score)	−.02	−.02	−.02
Married (M) Beta (depression)	−.10[c]	−.11[c]	−.09[c]
Beta (change score)	−.08[b]	−.08[c]	−.07[b]
Education (E) Beta (depression)	−.04	−.02	−.04
Beta (change score)	−.02	.01	−.02
Prior Income (I)			
Beta (depression)	−.11[c]	−.10[c]	−.11[c]
Beta (change score)	−.08[c]	−.07[b]	−.08[c]
Control			
W1 Distress			
Beta (change score)	.47[c]	.48[c]	.47[c]
Interactions [d]			
R x U Beta (depression)		−.03	
Beta (change score)		−.02	
E x U Beta (depression)		−.43	
Beta (change score)		−.65[c]	
F x U Beta (depression)		−.07	
Beta (change score)		−.07	
R^2(depression) =	.10	.10	.10
R^2(change score) =	.30	.31	.31

[a] Demographic data were obtained in Wave 1 except for marital status (Wave 3). N = 996.
[b] $p < .05$.
[c] $p < .01$.
[d] Interactions omitted because insignificant: A x U, B x U, B x I, B x E, and I x U (race models); A x U, B x F.
See text for race x marital status and race x seniority.

Models

We began as usual by testing for the main effects of unemployment and of each of the worker's personal characteristics, plus seniority (see Model I in Table 5.1). We followed this with one model to assess the "race package" of effects discussed earlier (Model II below) and one for the "gender package" (Model III). These latter models each added interactions to the first model—those that survived both initial testing by being entered separately into the model and testing in combinations. Given the reduced number of workers who were interviewed at Wave 3, we took several steps in an effort to minimize multicollinearity; this use of separate models for race and gender, in contrast to the omnibus approach at Wave 1, is an example. For race, we required that certain two–way interactions be significant. Then we examined the three–way interaction among race, education, and unemployment. As discussed below, this interaction cannot be tested reliably, with all the necessary demographic controls in this smaller Wave 3 data set. We can examine only the trends to see if they are consistent with the Wave 1 findings. We tested the race and gender models first without mediating and control variables, then adding financial hardship and negative life events. These mediated models are discussed later.

Analyses were always carried out for depression, anxiety, hostility, and somaticization. In general, patterns of response were similar across the four forms of distress; therefore we concentrate most heavily on depression. Where relevant, we also present results for anxiety, which generally paralleled depression.

THE LONG RUN: RESULTS

Table 5.1 summarizes what we found out about race, gender, unemployment, and depression. On the left, Model I includes only the main effects of each of the predictors. Results (standardized coefficients or betas) for Wave 3 depression scores are presented first; change scores appear beneath them. Because Model I includes only main effects, it is the baseline for more elaborate models for both race and gender. Model II (race) and Model III (gender) show the second stage in which we added two–way interactions, sequentially and in combination, to Model 1. A third round of modeling was done for race to test the three–way interaction (race–education–unemployment); as we have already alluded to, this analysis yielded estimates that were not necessarily reliable. For gender, no three–way relationship among gender, marital status, and unemployment was tested, given that no significant two–way interactions emerged. Two significant interactions involving race are omitted from Table 5.1 for parsimony. Race and marital status interacted in analyses that used raw distress scores, so that the effect of marital status on depression was greater for whites than for blacks. This paralleled the previously discussed gender–marital status pattern, in which the impact of marital status was greater for males than for females. It was also collinear with it, because blacks in our sample were more likely to be female than were whites. Because the race–marital status linkage was not predicted, we concentrate on the gender–marital status relationship (which was not significant by Wave 3). In addition, an unpredicted race–seniority interaction appeared in analyses of raw Wave 3 distress scores. Among whites, seniority had no relationship to distress, but higher seniority black workers tended to be more distressed. This was not a powerful trend, and it vanished when higher order interaction terms involving race and education were introduced.

Workers' Characteristics Revisited

As before, some workers were more likely to be distressed than others simply as a function of their personal characteristics, regardless of whether or not they were employed. We focus first on Model I in Table 5.1. Looking at the first coefficient for each predictor (i.e., that for Wave 3 depression), the table indicates that workers as of Wave 3 were at risk for depression simply for being (in rough order of the pervasiveness and strength of the effect):

female
of lower income initially
unmarried as of Wave 3
young

The two coefficients presented for each predictor are the results obtained for, first, Wave 3 depression and, second, change in depression between Wave 1 and Wave 3. Variables like gender, which have a powerful effect whether or not an event like unemployment occurs, have small and insignificant impacts on change across the panel study. Continuing the overview of Model I, black and white workers were essentially indistinguishable. In addition, although higher seniority workers reported significantly more symptoms as of Wave 3, as we mentioned earlier, this result was found only when accumulated unemployment was the independent variable (that is, cells b and d in Figure 5.1). Because Table 5.1 features cells a and c of Figure 5.1, we see no significant effect of seniority for either depression or change in depression. Finally, and most importantly, unemployment had effects everywhere. To be unemployed was to be more depressed and to have become more depressed over the course of the panel study.

Most evidence of vulnerability to the stress of unemployment concerned either race or gender as of Wave 1. Therefore in this analysis of Wave 3 distress, Model II focused on the former and Model III on the latter. In the language of Chapter One, both race and gender provide resources—capital—differentially. In general, blacks and women, relative to whites and men, tend to have fewer economic resources to provide immediate support during an economic crisis, and they may lack the human capital (e.g., education, experience) to make them attractive prospective employees. Next we turn to the way white versus black or male versus female can alter the meaning and the impact of unemployment.

Race. Model II shows, for both depression and change in depression, how two–way interactions in the "race package" affect distress. An education–unemployment interaction is significant for change in depression. Essentially a predictor like education–unemployment, which is dynamically related to distress over time, shows the opposite pattern to that we have seen for gender, and emerges in the analysis of change scores but not in the analysis of Wave 3 distress *per se*. The full three–way interaction, race–education–unemployment, also proved to be significant throughout the analyses carried out. Whether the issue was depression or change in depression and whether it was determined by unemployment or the accumulation/duration of unemployment, the same pattern as that seen at Wave 1 reappeared. Furthermore, it was evident across all the dependent variables (depression, anxiety, somaticization, and hostility). In one sense, this three–way relationship was a remarkably stable finding. In another sense, the small numbers of people represented in each of the combinations of characteristics meant that estimates of effect size for the race–education–unemployment interaction were likely to be unreliable.

In analyses not shown, the greatest distress appeared among unemployed, less educated, black workers. In addition, among blacks, education could be said to have a positive or protective mental health function that is not evident for whites. Among blacks with 12 or more years of education, unemployment did not have a negative impact on mental health, although it did for whites. In addition, the impact of unemployment is visible nearly everywhere; but just as it is smallest for the highly educated black workers, it is most severe for those black workers with less than 12 years' education. Black workers appear to be especially sensitive to their education levels—and, we presume, to the life chances that these educational levels make possible.

Gender. In thinking about gender, we first note that married females might be expected to have a resource advantage over males, based on marriage patterns. To assess this, we first considered whether females had working spouses more often than males, providing a kind of "insurance policy" against their own unemployment. Countervailing forces were at work in these data: Married women did more frequently have working spouses (by a margin of 77% to 55% at Wave 3), but male workers were more often married (by a margin of 80% to 39% at Wave 3). The overall rate at which workers had working spouses at Wave 3 was insignificantly higher for males (40%) than for females (35%). Other exploratory analyses (not shown) also indicated that the number of children did not have a significant impact on distress for either men or women; the number of children can be thought of as a form of resource drain.

With Marital Status. The impact of gender at Wave 3 depended somewhat on a worker's marital status and employment status, but the three–way interaction (gender, marital status, unemployment) was not significant. In fact, the two–way gender–marital status interaction that was significant at Wave 1 was only marginally so in the various regressions carried out for Wave 3. Comparsions of the mean scores, as done for Wave 1, still showed that the linkage between being married and having better mental health was true only among males (results not shown). Married males reported significantly fewer symptoms of depression than all other groups. Put another way, the average distress scores of married versus unmarried males differed significantly from one another, but the scores of married and unmarried females did not differ. Thus the same pattern was evident as in the earlier analysis of gender and marital status, although not powerfully enough to attain significance in the smaller Wave 3 sample and with all other predictors controlled.

Supplemental analyses using a more finely–tuned categorization of marital statuses (not shown here) also indicate that there was a progression in distress for men (married < cohabiting < widowed < single < divorced < separated), but for women a more detailed breakdown of marital status made no difference in their distress levels. For men, it mattered whether there was a woman around and why she had left; women showed no such sensitivity to the presence, absence, and departure of men.

With Unemployment. The gender–unemployment interaction was also insignificant for depression, as Model 3 illustrates—unless one considers the impact of accumulated unemployment on Wave 3 distress (results not shown). Because the latter analysis is the one discussed above as the one most likely to show results of all kinds, this is not a particularly powerful performance for gender. Nevertheless, this interaction was in the predicted direction: Men were more affected by unemployment than women. More persuasively, separate regressions for males versus females showed that the effect of unemployment was always larger for men than for women and was significantly different from zero only for the men. Looking at the results for Wave 3 depression, for men the effect of unemployment was significant (beta = .17, $p < .0001$; the effect for women was not (beta = .05). The same pattern emerges in Wave 2 (males, unemployment effect, beta = .17, $p < .0001$; females, unemployment effect, beta = .04, n.s.) and in Wave 1 (males, unemployment effect, beta = .07, $p < .05$; females, unemployment effect, beta = .01, n.s.).

Overall, these results indicate that gender specifies the linkage of unemployment to distress. There is a linkage, and it is significant for one group (men) and not for another (women); at the same time, these groups (the men and the women) may not differ significantly from one another. This is essentially a weak form of interaction. A specification requires only that one group's effect be different from zero and another group's not be; an interaction means that the two groups were significantly different from one another. On the whole, trends for the gender–unemployment connection were as expected, but the male–female gap in the effects of unemployment was of modest size.

Another way to illustrate the interplay of gender and unemployment is to examine and compare mean scores from an analysis of variance (ANOVA) (again using raw, unadjusted means).

Table 5.2 shows mean depression scores for each combination of gender and unemployment, plus marital status, at Wave 3. The literature suggests that the negative impact of unemployment should be particularly extreme among males, for whom the provider role might be threatened. Results are consistent with this expectation. Women did not differ significantly in mental health on the basis of their employment status. Men did. Put more globally, employed men differed significantly from all other groups, none of which differed among themselves.

In terms of the sheer statistics, a caution is in order. The three–way interaction of gender, marital status, and unemployment was not significant in regressions, regardless of whether we looked at depression or change in depression, and regardless of whether we examined the impact of Wave 3 or cumulative unemployment. But these analyses, like the ones for race and education and unemployment, faced a problem of potentially unreliable estimates because of the varying and sometimes small numbers of people in some combinations of gender, marital status, and unemployment; unreliability might suppress subtle findings. We are inclined to believe in the fact that certain specific contrasts (married employed men versus everyone else) were both significant and consistent with prior research.

In sum, results from the beginning and the end of our longitudinal study were quite consistent and straightforward. Depression was higher for women than for men, and it did not much matter whether the women had a job or didn't, has a husband or didn't. Among men, however, marriage mattered. Jobs mattered. And unemployment took a special toll on *married men*, relative to their mentally healthy starting point.

Although the findings involving gender, marital status, and unemployment are not powerful ones, they are consistent with a body of research on identity, gender, marital roles, and their interrelationship. To the extent that the mental health advantage of being male and, among males, the advantage of marriage, are each contingent upon the additional advantage of employment, there are special

Table 5.2

Gender and Marital Status as Contexts for Unemployment [a]

	Employed				Unemployed			
	Married		Unmarried		Married		Unmarried	
	Male	Female	Male	Female	Male	Female	Male	Female
N =	618	47	124	84	64	28	43	34
DEP [c]	1.35	1.67[b]	1.55	1.67	1.68	1.72	1.74	1.81
ANX [c]	1.24	1.54[b]	1.34	1.49[b]	1.47	1.56	1.48	1.58

[a] Wave 3 Unadjusted Means from 2 x 2 x 2 ANOVA. N = 1,042.
[b] Significantly different from the mean to its immediate left by post hoc Scheffe test at $p < .05$.
[c] DEP = depression and ANX = anxiety.

implications for males. However much the provider role offers mental health benefits to men when it is being fulfilled, it may also bring mental distress when it is not.

Given that these surveys did not include questions about various identities and their importance, it is not possible to test directly the importance of such identities as worker, husband, or their combination ("provider") (see Thoits, 1991; 1992). We shall return to the question of the provider role and its implications in discussing long–term stressors for men (i.e., combat). In the meantime, we can try to explain the results involving race and gender by means of mediating variables. Such an analysis need not conflict with an explanation in terms of identities and their importance; it may instead supplement it. Insofar as a mediating variable accounts for the impact of a variable like gender or gender in its interactions, it can be argued that the mediator in some sense captures what that variable or interaction means.

Mediators: Hardships and Events

Expectations about what might mediate the effects of gender and race are in part based on earlier summaries of workers' resources and hardships. Two factors are considered here: financial hardship and negative life events. We know from our earlier work that women experience more hardships (see chapter Three). Chapter Six will emphasize that hardships both lead to depression and account for the linkage of unemployment to depression. Therefore we expect women and blacks to experience more depression.

Another obvious possible difference between men and women, blacks and whites, concerns the other negative experiences life presents to them. Chapter Seven will consider in greater detail the measurement and meaning of "negative life events," as these experiences are usually termed. Here, the key questions concerned whether one or the other group (a) had experienced more negative life events (overall or of a particular type) and whether any group (b) was more vulnerable to the effects of some or all negative life events. Both the main effect of this index and its potential interaction with gender were assessed at each wave for each measure of distress.

Throughout the panel study, women reported significantly more negative life events than men, and blacks significantly more than whites. The key question concerns how these events impact on a person's distress levels. When we tested for the possibility that women or blacks might be differentially vulnerable to the impact of negative life events (i.e., that gender or race would interact with negative life events), we found no evidence that this was so. The true relationship was commonsensical: The more negative life events a worker had experienced in the previous year, the higher the depression (and anxiety, etc.). Therefore the potential impact of these life events rests on the fact that for women, and for blacks, life was more full of misery–generating happenings than it was for men, or whites. Again the syllogism is straightforward: Women/blacks experience more negative life events than men/whites; negative life events lead to distress; therefore we expect women and blacks to report higher levels of distress than men and whites. Such differences, like the differences in financial hardships, could themselves account for a much if not all of the "gender" or "race" differences thus far.

Results. Adding financial hardship and other negative life events to the models, the Model 2 equation left the results for race, education, the education–unemployment interaction—and (in the final equation) the race–education–unemployment interaction—still significant, although effects were generally reduced in size (results not shown). Essentially all that happened was we simply added two highly significant predictors to the equations. For example, in the analysis of Wave 3 depression for Model 2, the beta for financial hardship was .29 (p < .0001) and for negative life events was .27 (p < .0001). Similarly, results for W1–W3 change in depression included betas of .21 for hardship and .19 for negative life events (each p < .0001). Clearly, to experience hardship and to suffer through negative life events of whatever sort is to emerge more depressed. But whatever it is about being less educated, or black, or their combination, these new considerations do not change the story told about them earlier.

The story is different for gender. The beta for the effect of hardship was .29 in the Model III (gender) analysis of Wave 3 depression, and .21 for W1–W3 change. Corresponding betas for negative life events were .27, predicting Wave 3 depression and .19, predicting the W1–W3 change. (All betas were highly significant, p < .0001.) These effects were closely comparable in size to those found in analyzing race. However, with these mediators added to Model III, the gender–unemployment interaction and even the impact of gender itself were nil. Of course, the gender–unemployment interaction was not significant in the first place, except in equations including accumulated unemployment or in the form of specifications. The disappearance of gender itself from the significant predictors is impressive, however, especially for raw Wave 3 depression scores. The chapter's conclusions address what it may mean for gender to be "accounted for" by financial hardships and negative life events.

CONCLUSIONS

We all have to get through the day, even when life has dealt us a blow for which we were not prepared and for which we are not to blame. How do we do it? What keeps us going? Like Chapter Three, this chapter focused on the basic outlines of the mental health of the workers affected by the 1987 GM plant closings: who was hit, how hard they were hit, and something about their circumstances. Just as this chapter has concentrated on the "hard facts"—the social and economic circumstances that shape lives, that make it easier or harder to bear such burdens, Chapter Six focuses on the mechanisms by which unemployment has its effects. The approach throughout has been to think of human beings as bundles of resources. Resources can be concrete, like money (emphasized here). They can be interpersonal, like the support of loved ones (reviewed in Chapter Nine). And they can be psychological, like the person's way of looking at the situation (focused on in Chapter Eight), or memories (and scars) from events gone by (Chapter Seven). In general, a resource is anything a person can "spend" to help get out of or keep out of a mental health tailspin.

Race and Human Capital

What Chapter One labeled "human capital" variables, or "economic and cultural capital," emerged in this chapter as wellsprings of vulnerability to unemployment at the outset of the panel study. In the long run, this vulnerability faded somewhat. For example, prior income showed only a main effect on distress by Wave 3, and no longer increased vulnerability to mental distress in conjunction with unemployment. But education continued to alter the impact of unemployment on distress: Unemployment had more severe effects on mental health among less educated workers. These different trends for income and education make sense in terms of the fact that education, as cultural capital (Bordieu, 1986), can directly affect reemployment. Therefore, it may take on greater psychological importance over the long run. Throughout the study, race further modified the effect of education. Among the unemployed, black workers were particularly sensitive to educational levels. Less educated black workers were the most highly distressed, and more educated black workers were not appreciably distressed.

On balance, these variables, representing a kind of human capital model of workers' resources for combating stress, behaved in Wave 3 as they were expected to do and as they had done before. They affect workers' *overall levels* of distress, and also affect the *psychological impact of an economic stressor such as unemployment*. Human capital represents protection from financial crisis, and unemployment is first and foremost a financial crisis.

Gender and the Meaning of Unemployment

At both the beginning and the end of the panel study, gender interacted with marital status (Wave 1) or accumulated unemployment (Wave 3) to generate distress. Theoretically, we argued that these effects are part of a general complex of effects of gender, marital status, and unemployment in combination and that the impact of unemployment on various gender–marital status combinations is a function of the meaning to these workers of the roles they play. In particular, we noted that the biggest effect of unemployment is observed among married males, a finding which is consistent with their potentially holding a provider role in their families. Being male, which usually is associated with lower levels of depression and anxiety, can become a liability insofar as one of its key aspects—the subrole of "provider"—ceases to be fulfilled during a period of unemployment. Gender carries symbolic baggage, as well as economic implications. Gender *per se*, and the usual finding that women on average are more distressed than men, was easier to account for. The addition of two mediators—financial hardship and negative life events—eliminated the effects of gender *per se*. Interpreted literally, these results suggest that being a woman is generally associated with troubling events and persistent hardships; take those away, and a woman is no more distressed than a man. In general, the results suggest that gender plays a role in emotional life that is more than economic, and that aspects of either the male or the female gender role can be beneficial under some circumstances, and harmful under others. The emotional economy of gender is an economy of social and symbolic capital, as well as one of dollars and cents.

At the same time, it is plausible to be struck by how similar men and women were in their reactions to unemployment, rather than how different. We have previously noted that having a working spouse did not have different impacts on distress for men and women. These results—a pattern of subtle but significant trends that suggest the operation of gender roles—may be exactly what researchers should expect *when the comparison between men and women is made within class, within occupation, and within condition of current employment.* In contrast, to compare distress for employed males with distress for either housewives or females who work in quite different jobs is to load the dice in favor of finding "gender" effects. Precisely because what we know of "gender" *is* in large part a set of prescriptions about what people are supposed to do for a living and how they are supposed to do it. As Warr and Parry (1982) noted more than a decade ago, it is time to look at more precisely defined and specialized samples if we want to get a picture of what employment means to women psychologically.

Thoughts about Vulnerability

We have followed the conventional route by carrying out tests of whether unemployment affects mental health more sharply for one group than for another and by calling this difference *vulnerability*. Evidences of vulnerability to long–term unemployment, as shown here, however, can be interpreted in at least two ways. Take the recurring finding that unemployment affected distress more sharply for less educated workers. What does this mean? Either less educated workers are more hard hit psychologically by unemployment than other groups, or unemployment is an objectively worse stressor to them, or both. We suspect it is both.

The fact that we could not explain the education–unemployment interaction by taking into account two potent mediators—financial hardship and negative life events—is itself evidence for that interpretation. This failure may mean that we are looking to the past instead of the future. In the language of the life events literature, unemployment is both a major loss and a major threat. Therefore, workers who react to it, may be focusing both on what they have lost and on what they will have to face next. When education is viewed as cultural capital (Bordieu, 1986), the persistent impact of education throughout our study begins to look as if it reflects workers' look toward the future rather than the past.

The economic capital that attaches itself to people is a kind of "past tense" of stratification. Savings and wealth and personal income are examples. Unless they are large, they say less about future prospects than they do about yesterday's successes and the ability to pay one's bills today. Other resources, particularly those representing cultural capital, provide a "future tense," a promise of success to come. To lack cultural capital in a plant closing can give this event a different, much more crushing meaning. The concentration of misery among certain groups, such as the less educated in general, or less educated black workers specifically, might reflect their verdict on the future, not the past.

In a language closer to that of the workers themselves, conditions in Detroit or Flint, Michigan, in 1987–1990 can be thought of as a kind of macabre joke:

Q.: Where can a 40–year–old black guy with a 10th grade education get a job making $35,000 a year?

A: It just closed.

Sometimes it is just plain rational to be depressed.

6

A Question of Worth: Financial Circumstances, the Self, and Distress

Downsizing's most obvious consequence is financial. Whether job loss means financial inconvenience, struggle, hardship, or tragedy depends on the situation of the workforce as a whole and on individual workers' personal and family resources. Shutdown of a plant means a loss of livelihood for some, a threat to a way of life for others. Chapter One presented a model often used by sociologists to conceptualize the stressful aspects of unemployment; at the same time, we tried to highlight the ways in which autowork—a stable, unionized, well–paying blue–collar job—might generate thoughts, feelings, and concerns different from those experienced by either middle–class workers or the working poor. We noted that blue–collar workers seem to respond mainly to the financial implications of a shutdown, whereas middle class workers may be more likely to focus on psychological wounds such as the threat to identity that job loss represents. In contrast to the working poor, these autoworkers had the financial blow of job loss to some extent cushioned by factors as diverse as the supplemental unemployment benefits (SUB–pay) in the UAW–GM contract, the availability of outplacement assistance and job retraining, and the possibility of recall to their GM jobs when good times return (see discussion in Chapter Two). Potential job loss may have different meanings to blue–collar versus white–collar workers, to the unionized versus the nonunionized, and so forth. This chapter first examines one of the key ways in which unemployment appears to affect psychological well–being: the chapter explores how financial hardship affects mastery and self–esteem and how these in turn are linked to distress—especially depression. This is the natural order for these discussions because the stress model postulates that unemployment has effects both through hardship to distress, and through hardship to distress by way of the effects that financial hardship has on the psyche.

Part of what causes us to feel worthless is to be worth less. In many ways, this book can be seen as an exploration into the forms and meanings of worth: in the terms of Chapter One, forms of capital. Chapters Two through Four highlighted differences among workers in resources and experiences at the start of this plant closing study. Of the variants of capital discussed in Chapter One, economic capital has pervaded our discussions (Chapters Three, Five, and the current chapter). Human capital—what workers could do for themselves in the job market—was the focus of Chapter Five. This chapter's subject is the way in which issues of economic capital (financial worth) become issues of psychological capital (perceived hardship and self–worth) and how these in turn generate distress. Subsequent chapters will extend the discussion of capital to psychological as well as social capital. In Chapter Seven, a discussion of negative life events and prior stressors is intimately linked to the resource inequalities that lead some people to experience more such events and stressors. Psychological capital—how the worker thinks and feels about the self, how the worker plans for the future—is featured in Chapter Eight. Social capital—how the worker drew on social ties and contacts—is addressed in Chapter Nine.

FINANCIAL HARDSHIP

> When the layoff came along I still had all kinds of debts. Really, we didn't really know what was going to happen until just before they closed. When you have a family and a home and you're trying to get things together, you have loans and bills. I couldn't keep up on SUB–pay. My wife went to work but all she could get was minimum wage. So we lost our credit cards. We would have lost the house too, but my father stepped in and made us a loan to get caught up on the mortgage. Ever since the money troubles hit, my wife and I have had a love–hate relationship. We try, but all this causes trouble. It is just a lot of stress. This situation has certainly done us more harm than good.
>
> —a closing plant worker

Financial hardship actually plays three roles in the stress process: First, we know from Chapter Three that workers in closing plants are more often exposed to unemployment. If these workers are already more financially distressed than their counterparts in nonclosing plants before their jobs are lost, then it becomes difficult to make clear causal inferences about the effect of unemployment *per se.*

Unemployment falls on the shoulders of workers who are, inadvertently, "selected for" high initial hardship. Such problems involving the nonrandom distribution of characteristics are common in quasi–experimental designs, as Chapter Two discussed. Introducing statistical controls for initial financial differences is a key strategy to reduce this confounding of forces—one we use throughout the book. This chapter documents the need for this strategy by examining initial and later levels and types of financial hardship as they relate to employment status. Second, when workers are subjected to unemployment, financial hardship is clearly a major consequence. For blue–collar workers, the financial hardship caused may be *the* predominant effect of unemployment. Thus, financial hardship is a fundamental anticipated consequence of unemployment—a dependent variable—in a study like this. Third, in keeping with Chapter One's discussion of the life course and the stress process, we also ask how financial hardship serves to "translate" unemployment into such outcomes as depression or anxiety. Financial hardship is perhaps the major *intervening variable* by which unemployment shapes mental health. Its role can be thought of as fitting into a loose syllogism: Unemployment implies financial hardship; financial hardship implies distress; therefore unemployment implies distress. This chapter documents increases in financial hardship with unemployment and summarizes how financial hardship intervenes between unemployment and distress. As Chapter One suggested, hardship's influence on distress takes two paths. Hardship intervenes between unemployment and distress, and it influences the self–concept (mastery and self–esteem), which in turn affects distress.

Financial Resources

Financial resources are defined broadly to include both individual and familial resources; thus, savings and home ownership and having a working spouse can each be considered resources upon which the worker might draw. It is helpful to look at initial group differences in hardship and the effects of unemployment on hardship—the first and second questions above—in a single broad overview. The facts are straightforward. Wherever there were differences between closing and nonclosing plant workers or between the employed and the unemployed, as there almost always were, closing plant workers reported more hardships than nonclosing plant workers, and the unemployed more than the employed, in every wave of the survey.

Tables 6.1 and 6.2 indicate both the workers' initial and their final resource positions. Table 6.1 presents a series of indicators of financial well–being in terms of differences among closing plant workers who were already unemployed at Wave 1, closing plant workers who were vulnerable to unemployment, and nonclosing plant workers. All of the initial differences are significant. A look across the table from left (nonclosing plant workers) to right (already unemployed workers) reveals

Table 6.1
Workers' Wave 1 Financial Resources by Plant Type and Employment Status [a]

	Closing Unemployed	Closing Employed	Nonclosing
Hourly wage	9.22	13.17	13.85
Personal income (thousands)	34.7	39.8	43.5
Spouse works (% yes)	60.3	60.8	51.0
Family income (thousands)	35.5	41.1	45.1
Home owner (% yes)	55.5	78.5	91.1
Savings (% none)	19.2	16.0	12.1
Income declined (% yes)	n.a.	40.2	20.7
Financial hardship (percentile)	56.5	40.1	31.1

[a] Analyses were restricted to white and black workers who were not retired as of Wave 2 or Wave 3. N at Wave 3 ranged from 842 to 1,047 except for "spouse works," which was asked only of the married or cohabiting workers. All closing/nonclosing differences were highly significant at p < .01.

large gaps in financial status. Closing plant workers in general, and especially those already unemployed, report the following:
a lower hourly wage, lower personal income, and lower family income;
their spouses (usually wives) more often work;
they are less likely to own homes or have any savings;
*their incomes were already in decline from the previous year;
and their overall financial hardship (discussed below) is higher.
It is important to think of these numbers in the context of the rest of the American workforce. In that context, the picture of closing plant workers that emerges at the start of the study is one of relatively affluent people, but people living close to an edge. Most of them had incomes that put them financially in the

Table 6.2
Workers' Wave 3 Financial Resources by Employment Pattern [a]

	None	One	Two	Three
Hourly wage	15.2	10.9	7.8	0.0
Personal income (thousands)	38.6	18.2	11.0	9.0
Spouse works (% yes)	54.2	69.6	57.3	84.6
Family income (thousands)	46.4	27.7	21.0	20.1
Home owner (% yes)	90.0	72.2	76.5	66.6
Savings (% none)	6.9	24.1	31.3	45.8
Income declined (% yes)	20.1	44.5	57.1	40.7
Financial hardship (percentile)	29.5	50.6	58.9	69.1

Number of Times Unemployed

[a] Analyses were restricted to white and black workers who were not retired as of Wave 2 or Wave 3. N at Wave 3 ranged from 842 to 1,047 except for "spouse works," which was asked only of the married or cohabiting workers. All differences among groups based on unemployment patterns were highly significant at p < .01.

middle class. Their rate of home ownership exceeded the national average. But nearly one–fifth of them had no financial cushion ready when they fell, and they were heading for a fall.

Table 6.2 summarizes how several waves of unemployment can stretch out the resource difference between those who begin with more or fewer resources. We use a count of the "number of times unemployed" across the panel study to capture broad trends in the relationship of unemployment to financial hardship (see also Chapter Three). The worker who reports *none* for the number of times unemployed is highly likely to have started the study in the nonclosing plants; the worker who reports *three* for number of times unemployed must, by definition, have been in the closing plants (and among the initially unemployed within them). The general picture is one of widening gaps between groups. For example, whereas at the outset the unemployed closing plant workers already show a shocking 19.2% rate of having no savings at all, 45.8% of the three–times–unemployed workers reported at Wave 3 that they have no savings. Together, these tables show two aspects of financial hardship in relation to unemployment:

1. From the standpoint of statistics, there is a selection problem in this research, as we suspected. Workers who are "assigned" to unemployment by being in a closing plant are workers who lacked various financial resources *from the outset*. Life does not randomly assign unemployment but visits it upon those least able to handle its financial pressures.

2. Financial hardship is also an outgrowth of unemployment—a dependent variable—that is dynamic throughout a panel study like this.

Thus far, our evidence of financial hardship has been predominantly the "hard evidence" of such indicators as wages and income and savings. Stress, however, is in the eye of the beholder, and it is well known that events seen as highly stressful by some individuals are less stressful, or not stressful, to others (Lazarus & Folkman, 1984). The stress literature has evolved ways of measuring perceived hardship which we utilize. Conveniently, these questions overlap substantially the hardship items used in major studies of unemployment discussed in Chapter One, including Pearlin et al. (1981), Kessler et al. (1987a, b; 1988, 1989), and Caplan et al. (1989).

TRENDS IN FINANCIAL HARDSHIP

Workers who lack resources are likely to see themselves as hurting financially and to take concrete steps to deal with the hurt. Next, we take a concrete look at the ways in which workers saw themselves as financially hurting, and what, if anything, they attempted to do about that hurt.

Patterns of Hardship by Employment Status

Bills. The simplest summary of hardship as the worker saw it was the question of how hard it is to pay your bills. It is a question that everyone understands. How many workers found it "extremely difficult or impossible" to make monthly payments on their family bills, as the question put it?

As Figure 6.1 shows, the answer depends on how many times the worker reported being unemployed. Among the 688 workers who were never out of work, only 0.4% found it "extremely difficult or impossible" to pay their bills. Increasing percentages of these workers answered as the options moved to "very difficult," then "somewhat difficult," then "slightly difficult" (percentages not shown). Finally, over half (58%) responded that it was "not at all difficult" to pay their bills. Workers who had never lost jobs felt reasonably secure financially. They were not

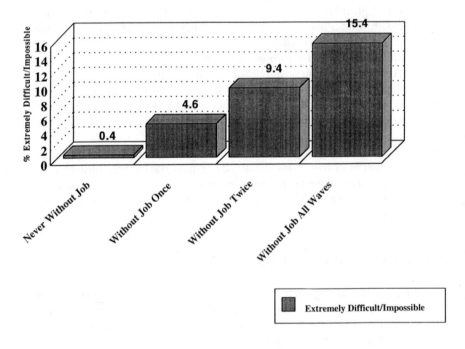

Figure 6.1. Employment status as predictor of difficulty paying bills in Wave 3.

as likely to be vulnerable to the kind of anxiety and shame of which we have spoken.

Workers who were not employed at any wave of the survey were not exactly the opposite of the always–employed, but close to it. More than 21% of them found it "extremely difficult or impossible" to pay their bills, and roughly equal numbers were distributed in each of the other categories. Not surprisingly, workers who were without a job once or twice gave roughly intermediate answers between those of the always–employed and the never–employed. Overall, the relationship between employment status and difficulty in paying bills is a powerful one that is quite unlikely to be a fluke of chance.

In thinking about what these numbers mean, we can see the glass as half–full or half–empty. On the one hand, lack of employment even across all three waves of the survey left some workers still able to get by. Fully 26% of those who never had a job claimed it was "not at all difficult" to pay their bills. On the other hand, this means that 74% experienced at least some difficulty, sometimes extreme. Lack of employment clearly translates into troubles with the mundane realities of keeping the family finances going. In evaluating the absolute size of this finding, we must also keep in mind the buffering that this workforce was provided by its benefits, as outlined in Chapter Two. Plants with no such safety nets—or even thin ones—can be expected to close with a more dramatic crash.

Basics. Ordinarily people who made more than $30,000 per year in 1987 would not be thought of as lacking money for food or medical care or clothing, let alone such items as leisure activities. But as our questions about ability to afford the basics showed, workers who lacked jobs felt the pinch even in these areas, even at the beginning of our study.

As Figure 6.2 illustrates, a stairstep pattern was evident by Wave 3: the more times without a job, the more difficulties. Predictably, all workers were more likely to report feeling a pinch on their leisure activities than in the areas of food or medical care or clothing purchases.

At the low extreme, less than 3% of those who were never without a job said that they "very often" or "fairly often" were not able to afford "the kind of food" they (or their family) should have. Similar percentages of these workers gave these same answers regarding "the kind of medical care" (2%) and "the kind of clothing" (3%) they or their family should have. Leisure activities were asked about a bit differently — the kind of leisure activities you/your family want (rather than "should have")— in such a way that perhaps invited more responses of deprivation. Of those never without a job, 8% reported being "very often" or "fairly often" unable to afford the leisure they wanted. Of course, this also means that fully 92% of this group was virtually always getting their leisure wants satisfied.

At the other extreme, at least 20% of the never–employed were "fairly often" or "very often" unable to afford each of the choices offered. Thirty–six percent

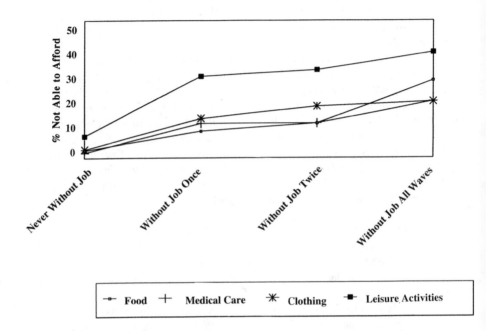

Figure 6.2. Employment status as a predictor of percentage "fairly often" or "very often" not able to afford.

could not afford food, 25% medical care, 25% clothing, and 43% leisure activities. The number for medical care is especially striking because workers retained their health care coverage for up to two years after their permanent layoff, so that coverage would have just been running out when they answered these questions—unless they had taken new jobs where the benefits were worse. Those who were out of work once or twice were, as before, intermediate between these extremes.

What do such numbers mean? Questions like these are standard ways of asking finances in surveys, but they have an obvious ambiguity. What does the food one's family "should have" mean? Does it mean avoiding starvation? Does it mean a balanced diet with all the food groups in the chart or circle or pyramid or whatever is in fashion? Does it mean serving Haagen–Daz instead of the generic store brand? We cannot be sure. We should not assume that workers and their families were literally deprived of food, but we can be confident that they felt deprived. And we can be certain that this feeling of deprivation was closely linked to the worker's pattern of employment.

Minor Hardships. The actions indicating minor hardships provide a window into what workers do when they feel financial pressure.

Table 6.3 summarizes how frequently workers in each employment category reported doing each action. The percentages refer to responses that the step had been taken "a great deal" or "quite a bit" and are arranged in descending order of their frequency among the group that was jobless at all waves.

It is important to keep in mind that in the third survey, as always, these questions referred to the "past 12 months." The previous two surveys, which asked the same questions, always showed differences between the jobless and the employed. To some extent, this stacks the deck against finding large differences among groups by our third survey. Looking at it from the worker's perspective, if you already cut back last year and had even started cutting back the year before that, will you respond that you cut back again? If you have already depleted your

Table 6.3

Wave 3 Employment Status as a Predictor of Minor Hardships in the Past 12 Months [a]

Percent saying "a great deal" or "quite a bit"

	Never Without Job %	Without Job Once %	Without Job Twice %	Without Job All Waves %
Cut back purchases	13.4	38.6	54.1	67.8
Decided not to buy planned purchase	11.4	30.2	36.8	35.7
Drawn more heavily from savings than usual	14.5	30.5	32.5	28.5
Postponed nonemergency medical or dental care because of cost	3.1	22.8	28.6	21.5
Borrowed money to help pay bills	2.4	9.0	8.3	21.4
Used credit cards or installment plans more than usual	6.0	16.3	15.9	17.8
Missed mortgage or rent payments	0.8	5.5	8.3	14.3
Missed other payments	1.0	7.4	7.6	14.3

[a] Items are arranged in order of descending frequency among those without work at all waves. Order of presentation in the survey is shown by the letter above each item. N ranged from 1,039 to 1,042. All chi–square tests were significant at p < .0001.

savings, how can you report that you drew extra money from savings? The sheer extent of hardship is probably underestimated here, simply because workers had already been dealing with financial troubles for a year or two.

Three messages emerge from this table regarding actions in response to hardship. First, the most noticeable difference across the groups is between those who were employed at all waves and everybody else. The always–employed were substantially less likely to respond that they had taken any of these actions with any frequency. Second, superimposed on this trend is the already familiar tendency for there to be a stepwise increase, a rising tide of hardship from the always–employed to the never–employed. Third, there are clear differences among the items. Some things people do quite readily. They cut back, they decide not to buy, they sneak a bit from savings. Other things they do more reluctantly. They postpone medical care. They borrow money so that they can pay bills, or (when they have them) they use credit cards to postpone the day of reckoning. Finally, they miss payments. Landlords and banks can take comfort that the last resort is to skip the rent or mortgage payment.

These data depict both a financial gulf and a slippery slide. The gulf is between those employed at all waves, for whom the most frequent action was drawing more heavily from savings, and everybody else. (A substantial percentage of the other groups either lacked savings in the first place or had already depleted them.) The slippery slide is from steady employment to steady lack of employment. At the extremes, the result is two financial worlds without overlap. The actions *least frequently* reported by those who were never employed (increasing use of credit cards, missing mortgage/rent, and missing other payments) were more common than the action *most frequently* reported by those who were always employed (drawing from savings).

Major Hardships. We asked about a standard roster of eight actions that indicate severe financial strain, but we found that a couple — "looked for a new job" and "refinanced mortgage" — did not add much to our understanding of the impact of the plant closings. In every survey, those who were not employed were more likely to be looking for a job. So all "looked for a new job" really tells us is that a plant closing means jobs are lost and people who don't have jobs look for jobs. The question about mortgage refinancing was problematic for other reasons. First, as we have seen, workers from nonclosing plants were more likely to have mortgages that they *could* refinance. Second, mortgage refinancing was occurring relatively frequently during this period in response to dropping interest rates, so that having refinanced a mortgage did not necessarily indicate any financial hardship at all. In fact, this item did not show any particular relationship to employment patterns.

The six additional items in this group seemed more likely to reveal real information about severe hardship: "used Medicare/Medicaid," "used food stamps," "used public assistance (welfare)," "used rent/heat subsidy," "moved to lower payments," and "pawned or sold items."

For the most part, Table 6.4 indicates that these questions produced the same pattern of difference among employment groups as those shown in Table 6.3. Never being without a job was the best of worlds, and never having one was the worst of worlds. But the level of extreme distress was not high. Among those who were without jobs at all three waves, the most frequent "yes" response concerned Medicare/Medicaid, and only 18% reported that they made use of either. This is in keeping with the fact that these workers had started out with relatively well–paying jobs and their union contract provided a safety net of pay and benefits.

Children's Hardships. For a worker with children, one particularly painful aspect of a plant closing is the hardship it brings to these small victims of the crisis. Seven questions asked about the hardships that might be felt by children aged 5–22 (an age range chosen because it encompasses school and college activities and attendance).

Although the number of workers who responded was naturally smaller, Table 6.5 shows that for questions about younger children (5–16), exactly the same pattern of differences among employment groups still held. Workers who were never without a job were distinctively different from all others, hardly ever having to deprive their children of activities, lessons, clubs, or camps. The more times the worker was without a job, the more the children suffered.

For older children, these differences were muted or absent. We asked whether children in the 16–22 range had to quit or change their schooling because of money and whether they had started to work to earn money. In neither case were differences evident at any wave of the survey, whether based on workers' plant closing status, employment status, or cumulative employment status. It is possible that these questions were not fully appropriate to this blue–collar work force,

Table 6.4

Employment Pattern as Predictor of Actions Indicating
Major Financial Hardship at Wave 3 [a]

	Never Without Job %	Without Job Once %	Without Job Twice %	Without Job All Waves %
Used Medicare/Medicaid	2.2	5.9	9.8	17.9
Used food stamps	0.4	5.9	9.0	17.9
Used public assistance	0.6	3.0	9.8	14.3
Used rent/heat subsidy	0.9	2.0	10.5	10.7
Moved to lower payments	0.6	5.4	6.8	3.6
Pawned or sold items	3.1	13.9	18.8	3.6

[a] Items are arranged in order of descending frequency among those without work at all waves. Order of presentation in the survey is shown by the letter above each item. N ranged from 1,041 to 1,044. All chi–square tests were significant at p < .0001.

whose children may not be college–bound and who may feel that the purpose of *anyone* going to work is to earn money. (This latter point is supported by the startlingly high percentages of employed workers who said in each survey that their older children had started to work to earn money — more than 70%, which is similar to the percentage for those without work.)

Therefore, the overall picture of hardships experienced by children is less clear than the picture for their parents. We can be relatively sure that younger children suffered real cutbacks, but we cannot be sure about whether their older brothers and sisters did. More importantly, the combination of answers to these questions about hardships can be read as a real attempt to protect the children. Quite simply, the numbers in Table 6.3 tend to be larger than those in Table 6.5. (Of course, the first of these tables refers to all workers, whereas the second refers only to those workers with children. However, when we reexamine the figures in Table 6.3 only for workers with children, the patterns remain the same as before.) Regardless of their employment status, workers were less willing to cut back on sending their children to the movies, for example, than on purchases as a whole. When workers and their families were faced with real hardship, this could lead to troubling choices and financially risky decisions. For example, at Wave 3 a larger proportion of those who were consistently out of work were skipping mortgage or rent payments than were denying their children summer camp. Children were clearly affected by their parents' job turmoil. But they were also protected.

Table 6.5
Percentage of Workers Whose Children Had to Limit Activities [a]

	Never Without Job %	Without Job Once %	Without Job Twice %	Without Job All Waves %
Free time activities (e.g., movies)	7.7	19.0	28.4	33.3
Lessons outside school	3.3	13.9	16.7	11.8
Other clubs/groups (Boy Scouts, church, etc.)	1.8	9.0	13.6	11.1
School activities, clubs	2.0	10.0	14.9	12.5
Summer camp	1.6	8.9	20.9	5.9

[a] N ranged from 646 to 651. Items were asked only of those workers who had children aged 5–22. All chi–square tests were significant at p < .0001.

FINANCIAL HARDSHIP AS PART OF THE STRESS PROCESS

Predicting Financial Hardship

What really affects financial hardship? Preexisting roles, groups, and identities? Losing a job? Their combination? In several places we have suggested—and shown—that certain social roles and social facts are linked to financial hardship. Now we can take a final look at financial hardship as a dependent variable by regressing perceived hardship on the standard demographic factors considered throughout the book (race, gender, marital status, education, seniority, age, and prior income) and on employment status. To be relatively conservative, we try to explain financial hardship at Wave 3 by unemployment at Wave 3, rather than an accumulation of unemployment.

Table 6.6 presents an omnibus analysis of financial hardship as part of the stress process; it is a table to which we shall return repeatedly through the chapter, but now we concentrate on the question of what predicted financial hardship: the first column of data on the left. Results for the previous two waves were also checked and found quite similar.

Table 6.6
Inside the Stress Model: Predicting Change in Depression (W1–W3) [a]

	Financial Hardship	Mastery	Self–Esteem	Change in Depression
Seniority	−.20	−.002	−.002	.002
Race (1=black)	1.57	.06	.03	−.05
Gender (1=female)	6.08[b]	.05	.03	.04
Marital Status (1=married)	.20	−.04	.03	−.06
Age (years)	−.82	−.01[c]	.002	−.002
Education (1=12+)	−2.70[c]	.10[b]	.04	.01
Prior Income (thousands)	−.34[c]	.004[c]	.002[c]	.00
Wave 3 Unemployment (1=unemp.)	17.48[c]	−.10[b]	−.01	.05
Negative Life Events (W2–W3)	5.03[c]	−.05[c]	−.00	.07[c]
Financial Hardship W2–W3	——	−.005[c]	−.001[c]	.002[c]
Mastery	——	——	.38[c]	−.21[c]
Self–Esteem	——	——	——	−.48[c]
Depression Wave 1	——	——	——	.24[c]
Constant	44.20	3.87	2.27	3.54
$R^2 =$	.54	.15	.36	.54

[a] N = 990.
[b] $p < .05$.
[c] $p < .01$.

When all the predictors of hardship are pitted against one another, logic prevails. Economic capital and the wherewithal to get it should be and are the major predictors: here, they are represented by prior income and current employment status. Also important are education, which provides human capital, and negative life events other than unemployment itself. Many negative life events have indirect implications for finances or are even the results of changes of fortune. For example, divorce or death of a spouse may have serious financial implications.

In "explaining" financial hardships through such things as the negative events that occur to people, we must also remember that the direction of causation can go two ways. Just as negative events can generate hardship, the occurrence of financial hardships can precipitate negative life events (e.g., moving to a worse neighborhood, marital separation). Almost certainly, both of these flows of influence occur.

For present purposes, we were most interested in seeing which of the "classic" demographic predictors—race, gender, age, marital status—were related to financial hardship *when economic factors were controlled.* The answer is straightforward: gender. Controlling for race, age, seniority, education, and marital status and taking into account several of the ways in which women were disadvantaged relative to men (lower income, higher unemployment, and more additional negative life events), women still reported greater financial hardship than men.

Overall, the main message of this first column of Table 6.6 is clear: to lack money, jobs, and/or skills is to experience financial hardship. And to be female has its own, separate costs.

Accounting for the Impact of Unemployment

The logic by which financial hardship enters into the stress process is straightforward. If unemployment affects distress because people are financially deprived, then it should be possible to take any given relationship between unemployment and distress, add financial hardship to the equation, and find that the effect of unemployment is largely if not entirely accounted for. This is precisely the argument in Pearlin et al.'s (1981) testing of the stress model. Similarly, Kessler et al. (1987a, b) found that in a blue–collar sample, financial hardship (measured quite similarly to our own indicator) accounted for about half of the impact of unemployment on mental health. Next we assess whether our findings with blue–collar workers fit well or poorly with the conclusions of these prior studies.

Table 6.7 summarizes the relationship of unemployment and financial hardship as predictors of depression for each wave of the study. Results are expressed in terms of standardized as well as unstandardized coefficients in this table to facilitate two kinds of comparisons. The standardized coefficients (b) are in the same metric and allow the reader to make direct comparisons (here, between unemployment and financial hardship). The unstandardized coefficients (B) allow the reader to see how big a change in the dependent variable (depression) is caused by a change of one unit in the independent variables. Here, because unemployment is a dichotomy (employed/unemployed), a change of one unit is a maximum change; because financial hardship is a percentile, many finer gradations of change exist. This means that unstandardized coefficients for these two variables are likely to be quite different, even if their predictive strength is the same.

For each wave of the survey, the column entitled "Model I" in Table 6.7 presents the simple univariate relationship between unemployment and depression. The column entitled "Model II" shows what happens when financial hardship is added to the equation. Table 6.6 has already displayed the end product of this mediation process; its far right column shows that financial hardship is a substantially more powerful predictor of depression than unemployment. Table 6.7 simply provides the details of how much financial hardship matters. In Waves 1 and 2 of the survey, unemployment is no longer significant when financial hardship is taken into account. In Wave 3, unemployment remains significant but its effect is substantially smaller. Overall, financial hardship accounts for nine–tenths of the variation in depression that is associated with unemployment at Wave 1; four–fifths of the Wave 2 variation; and more than half of the variation in Wave 3. In addition, financial hardship appears to be a kind of "value added" intervening variable. It does more than just account for the effect of unemployment; it adds dramatically to the ability to explain depression. Explained variance (R^2) goes up from about 1% to nearly 20%.

Table 6.7

Financial Hardship as Mediator of Unemployment–Depression Relationship [a]

	Model I Direct Effect		Model II Mediated Effect	
	b	B	b	B
Wave 1				
Unemployment	$.20^b$	.10	.01	.01
Financial hardship	n.a.		$.009^b$	.39
Wave 2				
Unemployment	$.28^b$	.20	.06	.04
Financial hardship	n.a.		$.007^b$	.37
Wave 3				
Unemployment	$.30^b$	.20	$.12^b$	$.08^b$
Financial hardship	n.a.		$.007^b$	$.38^b$

[a] Standardized coefficients are to the right of the unstandardized coefficients. Regressions were restricted to workers who had data at all three waves. N's ranged from 1,032 to 1,042.
[b] Effect significant at $p < .01$.

These results are consistent with previous findings about the importance of financial hardship as a consequence of unemployment. They also suggest that we should further explore the powerful linkage of financial hardship to distress. The next section of this chapter does so by introducing two important elements of self–concept—mastery and self–esteem—as intervening between financial hardship and distress in the stress process. In the model of Figure 1.1, these self–related variables were pictured as caused by unemployment and financial hardship, and in turn causing distress. They are pivotal indicators of whether and to what extent financial "worth less" becomes personal "worthless."

CONCLUSIONS I: FINANCIAL WORTH

Closing plant workers were in consistently greater financial difficulty than nonclosing plant workers, and some of their hardships grew over time. There was a systematic relationship between the number of times a worker was out of work and the financial hardships experienced. Only the steadily employed escaped financial threat. Within closing plants, hardships were fewer among those workers who managed to stay employed or get reemployed, but they were still significant—regardless of the worker's race, gender, age, marital status, or seniority. At the extreme, then, experienced white, male, GM workers whose plant closed down could expect financial troubles compared with workers in nonclosing plants, even if they managed to stay employed—unless they could stay with GM.

Financial hardship is also implicated as an important mechanism by which unemployment leads to distress, such as the depression symptoms examined here. As we argued at the start of this chapter, financial hardships play a multifaceted role in stress experienced by the unemployed:

1. Hardships differentiate workers such that those in greater initial hardship are more likely to experience unemployment.

2. Hardships grow over time in response to unemployment.

3. Hardships serve as the intervening variable through which unemployment is associated with distress.

It is also important to assess these findings in the light of this study's limitations. Although we have seen repeated evidence of significant impacts of unemployment on the financial lives of these workers and their families, this evidence probably understates the case in terms of the larger picture of downsizing and unemployment in America. The combination of income protection programs and continued benefits available to most UAW members throughout the period of our study may make "unemployment" mean something different for these workers — something less stressful -- than would be true in a workforce not protected by a union. However serious, the hardships caused by the 1987 GM plant closings are likely to be less extreme than those typically encountered when a blue–collar job is lost.

PSYCHOLOGICAL WORTH

What has it done to me? Well, lately, I guess you could say
I'm having a midlife crisis or something. This has all been
kind of a loss of stature—you feel kind of worthless. I don't
see anybody from the old plant—we just don't even want
to see each other. I can't even drive by the place. It sort
of tugs on the heart. I stay at home most of the time. Social
life? Huh, there isn't one anymore. I don't know what is going
to happen. I just try to hang in there.

–a closing plant worker

The self is both a social product—an effect—and a social force, a cause (Rosenberg, 1981). As Chapter One noted, bringing the self into the study of stress and distress can contribute to the evolution of a more comprehensive model of stress through the life course (Elder, 1994). In the stress process, an event like job loss has effects on the psyche and not solely on the purse. Specifically, the Pearlin et al. (1981) model of the stress process featured mastery and self–esteem as overarching psychological constructs that might stand between unemployment (or more broadly, financial hardship) and distress and hence mediate their relationship. This chapter pursues this line of reasoning.

Our analysis is somewhat abbreviated by the constraints on what we asked workers and when. Because interview time was constrained and there were multiple demands that we ask items of various sorts, these psychological variables were asked only late in the panel study. Measures of mastery and self–esteem were asked of closing plant workers in the second wave of the panel survey, one year after the plants closed, but were available only for the entire data set in the third wave of the survey. Therefore, it is not feasible to analyze change scores over the whole survey, as we do in other places.

For the most part, analyses will follow the same logic followed for financial hardship:

1. First, we think of mastery and self–esteem as dependent variables: In what ways are they directly affected by workers' characteristics or by unemployment?
2. Second, does either mastery or self–esteem serve as a mediator between unemployment and the distress that follows? That is, does a person's sense of mastery or self–esteem serve to filter and channel and give meaning to job loss?
3. Third, how are the effects of these aspects of the self altered by other factors

(moderators)?

One particular type of moderator is the effect of prior stressors upon current stress processes via the self. Elements of self, once shaped by social life, can play an active role in a person's subsequent experiences, including stressful ones.

For the most part this portion of the chapter compares workers at Wave 3 on the basis of current employment versus joblessness. As Chapter Five noted, this is relatively conservative in that we pick up only current costs of unemployment and do not tap longer term legacies (e.g., from persistent unemployment). The final dependent variable is distress as of Wave 3, taking mastery and self–esteem into account as predictors of distress, but without controlling for a worker's initial levels of mastery or self–esteem. Thus, we can not take advantage of the study's longitudinal design to clarify causal inferences; however, the entire sample is included, instead of restricting the analysis to the closing plant workers (who responded to questions about mastery and self–esteem in two waves of the survey). To be able to cross over from one survey to another helps in ruling out reverse causation; one variable taken from an earlier survey cannot be caused by a second variable taken from a later one. In this context, it should be remembered that most survey research is cross–sectional. It was the difficulty of causal inference in such circumstances that spurred the development of causal modeling. Like most survey researchers, we will be asking questions about whether the model we use is plausible, whether it is theoretically justified, and whether it fits the data well, but we will not be able to take advantage of the dynamic (panel) nature of the data.

Analyses of mastery and self–esteem as dependent variables and as intervening in the stress process each build upon and add to the analyses that come before. The same personal characteristics (race, gender, age, and the like) are always taken into account. The other negative life events experienced by the worker during the previous year are always taken into account; and as the first half of this chapter suggested, financial hardships experienced are also included in our models. We move, as in the first chapter's figures, from a person's past and enduring traits to the current crisis of employment to the burden of hardships it brings on, keeping in mind the other crises that may be occurring. In the stress model, mastery and self–esteem simply occupy the next step on the way toward distressed mental health.

Descriptive Statistics

Differences. The basic differences—or the lack of differences—in workers' sense of mastery on the basis of demographic characteristics that were categorical in nature (race, gender, education, and marital status) were as follows. Mastery was significantly related only to education, and more highly educated workers were higher in the sense of mastery. Gender approached significance, and men reported greater mastery. There were parallel findings for self–esteem. More educated and married workers were significantly higher in self–esteem. The lack of difference in self–esteem between the races might seem surprising, but in fact black children, adolescents, and adults tend to score equal to or higher than their white counterparts (e.g., Broman et al., 1989; Rosenberg, 1979). It is noteworthy that the determinants of these two highly correlated aspects of self are not identical, and self–esteem is predicted by a larger number of the workers' personal characteristics.

We also assessed the relationships of mastery and self–esteem to the continuous predictors, seniority, age, and income. Because these are continuous variables, results can be expressed correlationally. Mastery was negatively related to seniority ($r=-.06$, $p=.04$) and to age ($r=-.12$, $p<.0001$), but correlated positively with the worker's prior income ($r=.14$, $p<.0001$). Self–esteem was also positively linked to income ($r=.18$, $p<.0001$) but was unrelated to seniority or age.

Predicting Mastery and Self–Esteem

Next we carried out regressions in which all demographic variables plus relevant other predictors (unemployment, financial hardship, negative life events) predicted mastery and self–esteem. These results appear in the second and third columns of Table 6.6. When all predictors were taken into account, the linkage between seniority and mastery (with high seniority linked to low mastery) was no longer significant. This probably reflects the fact that age, which was highly correlated with both seniority and a stronger predictor of mastery, was included along with seniority. Three demographic factors significantly predicted mastery in this regression: educational level, age, and prior income. (More educated, younger, and higher income workers reported higher mastery.) In addition, unemployment, financial hardship, and negative life events were each associated with lower mastery.

The parallel regression for self–esteem reconfirmed the importance of prior income as related to self–esteem, and financial hardship was added to the list of significant predictors. In contrast, neither education nor marital status was significant when other demographics were taken into account. This need not mean that these variables are without impact. For example, there is a possibility of indirect causation; perhaps a high level of education leads to mastery which leads to self–esteem.

Theoretically, it is important that mastery is treated as a predictor of self–esteem in Table 6.6. Empirically, the two concepts correlate highly; it can be thought of as a matter of choice whether to treat them as two parts of a single thing, to treat mastery as the driving force, to pick self–esteem for that role, or to conceptualize the relationship as one of reciprocal causation. As Chapter One suggested, we believe that in the adult, mastery and self–esteem are constantly influencing one another. They cause one another. But in human development, mastery is temporally prior to self–esteem. A sense of mastery is built from experience; a sense of self–esteem, in turn, is built upon the perception that one has a separate and efficacious self (see Bandura, 1977, 1995; Rosenberg, 1981). Further, in adult life mastery is more labile, more experience–driven, more likely to respond to crisis with change. Therefore, to simplify our model, we give mastery causal priority.

Just as the relationship of mastery to self–esteem cannot be taken for granted, the impact of demographic factors need not invariably "cause" psychological factors. In the case of race or gender, the assumption of one–directional causation is correct. Because both are relatively fixed and immutable, it is gender/race that causes self–esteem and not the reverse. (We recognize that such is not impossible, e.g. racial "passing" or transsexual operations do occur, and in both directions). In the case of other demographic variables, however, the relationship is less clear. And it is those other, less firmly fixed demographic factors that relate to mastery and/or self–esteem. To be educated or to have higher income builds mastery; high income builds self–esteem; but it is also plausible that those who possess greater self–esteem and who feel greater mastery would go on to higher levels of education or have higher earnings. Although we occasionally fall victim to our belief that certain demographic facts cause certain psychological ones, all we can firmly establish is the existence of linkages between them.

Effects of Unemployment. Table 6.8 summarizes the comparisons involving unemployment for both mastery and self–esteem, overall and within closing plants. Analyses are restricted to workers who were not retired and who were either white or black. Trends over time appear for the closing plant workers alone, because only they responded to these questions at both Waves 2 and 3. The first comparison in the table shows that both mastery and self–esteem rose significantly between Wave 2 and Wave 3. Remembering that peak unemployment occurred at Wave 2—and half of closing plant workers were jobless—one obvious possibility is that the sense of mastery and self–esteem rose among those who got jobs.

For this reason, the middle of Table 6.8 shows comparisons between the employed and unemployed closing plant workers as of each wave. At Wave 2, these groups do not differ significantly in their sense of mastery, and self–esteem differences, although statistically significant, are small. By Wave 3, however, the usual and predictable relationship between employment and self–concept emerges. Employed closing plant workers are significantly higher in both mastery and self–esteem than their unemployed counterparts. The lower section of the table shows results for the entire sample, nonclosing as well as closing plant workers; the picture of the impact of unemployment which emerges is virtually identical to that suggested in the middle panel. This is in part due to the stable job–holding of workers whose plants did not close; they remained employed and remained at GM.

Returning to the middle of Table 6.8, one common pattern emerges for mastery and self–esteem: Scores of the unemployed are virtually identical from one wave to the next. It is the scores of employed workers that rise by Wave 3, producing the

Table 6.8
Effects of Time and Unemployment on Self–Esteem and Mastery [a]

	Mastery	Self–Esteem
Time (closing plants only)		
Wave 2 vs.	.28[d]	3.63[d]
Wave 3 [b]	3.40	3.69
Unemployment: (closing plants)		
Wave 2 employed vs.	3.34	3.66[c]
Wave 2 unemployed	3.21	3.62
Wave 3 employed vs.	3.47[d]	3.72[d]
Wave 3 unemployed	3.25	3.61
Unemployment: full sample		
Wave 3 employed vs.	3.45[d]	3.73[d]
Wave 3 unemployed	3.24	3.60

[a] N = 1,046 for the full sample.
[b] a) In comparison, Wave 3 grand means (closing plus nonclosing plants) were self–esteem=3.71, mastery=3.42.
[c] $p < .05$.
[d] $p < .01$.

significant differences over time shown above. There are at least two reasons that this might be the case. One involves the newly reemployed worker. This is a person who it is easy to imagine, gains in the sense of control and feelings of self–worth. If "employed" as a category has a larger number and percentage of these newly re–employed workers by Wave 3, then scores would rise as we see here. A complementary explanation might involve closing plant workers who remained employed from Wave 2 to Wave 3. Chapter Three emphasized that a considerable number—half—of the workers in the closing plants did not lose jobs. But they probably lost sleep. Indeed, Chapter Four showed that even nonclosing plant workers had elevated anxiety at the outset of our study. How much more anxiety and other distress might be generated in those who still work the line, watching their friends and co–workers depart? The benefits of employment may well be tempered by a fear that "there but for the grace of God go I."

The lack of difference seen at Wave 2 between closing plant workers who did and did not have jobs can be understood in terms of both the forces that distinguished employment from unemployment more starkly at Wave 3 (reemployment), and, conversely, the forces that made employment resemble unemployment more closely at Wave 2 (fear of job loss). We will explore patterns in employment status at greater length in Chapter Eight, whose primary concern is the role of psychological resources. These include what people think or expect of their job situation.

MASTERY AND SELF–ESTEEM IN THE STRESS PROCESS

Chapter One's theoretical model of the stress process argued for the possibility that a stressor like unemployment has effects on mental health through its financial effects and through the impact that unemployment and financial hardship have on views of the self. The previous literature has emphasized the roles of mastery and self–esteem. To be an intervening variable that stands between stress and its consequences, mastery or self–esteem, like financial hardship earlier in this chapter, must play a dual role. It is a dependent variable with regard to demographic factors, unemployment, and other important controls such as Chapter Six's negative life events. Mastery and self–esteem can also be dependent variables with regard to financial hardship. This is captured visually in the fact that they stand to its right in the figures of Chapter One.

A final question about the way mastery and self–esteem are generated concerns the relationship between the two psychological constructs themselves. Because of the limited data available, we can argue, but not prove the theoretical position we will take, that mastery causes self–esteem, whereas either or both of them may be related to distressed mental health. This is why Figure 1.5 showed arrows from financial hardship to both mastery and self–esteem, from mastery to self–esteem, and then from both to depression. Now it is time to make the first leg of this causal journey by asking what accounts for mastery and self–esteem.

Returning to Table 6.6 and moving from the left (financial hardship) to the right, the results of equations that predict first mastery, then self–esteem, and finally Wave 1–Wave 3 change in depression appear. Again we emphasize that depression is a consequence of unemployment because unemployment has its most potent and longest lasting influence there; results for anxiety and hostility will be reported later. The change in depression rather than the raw depression score is selected as the dependent variable because it gives us a relatively conservative estimate of the effect of joblessness that is focused on the period of the plant closings (see also Chapter Five). Controls always include age, race, education, prior income, and other negative life events. Because age and seniority were highly collinear in these analyses, we used age rather than seniority, which is more generally relevant. The initial dependent variable (financial hardship) is a predictor in all equations to its right and so forth: Mastery predicts self–esteem and depression, whereas self–esteem predicts depression.

Significant predictors of change in depression between Wave 1 and Wave 3 included financial hardship, negative life events, mastery, self–esteem, and the Wave 1 level of depression. One thing about this list is noteworthy: There are no objective demographic predictors whatsoever. No race, no gender, no marital status, no age, no education, no income, no unemployment. And yet, we have seen such linkages throughout this book; Chapter Five, in particular, is devoted to the impact of workers' own characteristics. Then what is happening? We are witnessing evidence of success, success in getting inside the stress model to specify how objective predictors lead to distress. For example, now we know that unemployment leads to depression by the following paths:

Unemployment leads to financial hardship.
Financial hardship leads to loss of mastery.
Financial hardship leads to loss of self–esteem.
Loss of mastery leads to loss of self–esteem.

Financial hardship, low mastery, and lack of self–esteem lead to distress.

And sometimes unemployment still has its own unique contribution to make to distress (see the next discussion of the stress process among men).

This does not mean that unemployment is unimportant for depression. On the contrary, it means that the effects of unemployment are ubiquitous.

Anxiety and Hostility

Table 6.9 presents results of the same series of models as Table 6.6, simply substituting anxiety or hostility for depression. The only columns that are needed are the final ones, showing what affected the two distress measures, because everything before that in the models—predicting financial hardship, mastery, and self–esteem—is unchanged. For the most part the same things that lead to anxiety and hostility lead to depression. One factor, age, uniquely predicts hostility. Younger people may feel, express, or enact greater hostility than their older counterparts. The evidence here refers only to their willingness to express hostile feelings.

One factor in Table 6.9, financial hardship, fails to predict anxiety. This is not because financial hardship is unimportant in generating anxiety; instead, further examination of the patterns of results shows that financial hardship's effect on anxiety is mediated by mastery. This makes sense in terms of Chapter One's discussion of the stress process. Anxiety should generate a reduced sense of mastery and vice versa; fear and loss of control go hand in hand. Thus, if financial hardship generates anxiety—which it does—we may be able to capture the essence of that relationship if we control for mastery. Here, we were able to do so. Ultimately, such a relationship is circular:

Financial hardship affects mastery.
Financial hardship affects anxiety.
Mastery affects anxiety.
Anxiety affects mastery.
Mastery affects the ability to hold a job.
Employment affects financial hardship.

Table 6.9 cuts into this circle at a particular point.

Table 6.9
Mastery and Self–Esteem as Mediators:
Predicting W1–W3 Change in Anxiety and Hostility [a]

	Change in Anxiety	Change in Hostility
Seniority	.002	.003
Race (1=black)	−.00	−.05
Gender (1=female)	.08	−.00
Marital status (1=married)	.00	.04
Age (years)	−.00	−.006[c]
Education (1=12+)	−.03	.00
Prior income (thousands)	−.001	.00
Wave 3 unemployment (1=unemp.)	.04	−.03
Negative life events (W2–W3)	.02[b]	.04[c]
Financial hardship W2–W3	.00	.002[c]
Mastery	−.16[c]	−.16[c]
Self–Esteem	−.35[c]	−.33[c]
Wave 1 distress	.27[c]	.25[c]
Constant	2.78	2.89
$R^2 =$	.37	.34

[a] N = 990.
[b] $p < .05$.
[c] $p < .01$.

Moderators: Race, Gender, and the Self

Thus far we have demonstrated intimate linkages between self—mastery and self–esteem—and distress: depression, anxiety, and hostility. It appears that Chapter Five's approach to explaining distress, emphasizing demographic factors that might serve as resources for combating stress, is incomplete. Referring to Chapter Five raises a question, however, about the role of certain demographic factors as they may affect the self. Specifically, Chapter Five showed that *race* and *education* interacted with unemployment to produce a particular vulnerability among blacks with less than high school educations. Also, gender interacted with unemployment (and to some extent gender, marital status, and unemployment interacted) so that men were more affected by unemployment than women, and the impact of unemployment was most pronounced among married men. If this is true of forms of distress like depression, might it also be so for mastery or self–esteem?

Race. We addressed the question of the relationships of race and education, together with unemployment, to mastery and for the gender–unemployment link. These relationships were significant only for mastery. It should be emphasized that the race–education–unemployment relationship was marginal (p = .07), and there were no significant interactions involving gender, unemployment, and/or marital status.

There was also no evidence that self–esteem was linked to either race or gender in an interactive relationship.

What is interesting about the findings is their similarity to the depression results reported in Chapter Five. Throughout the three waves of the study, we found that depression fell especially hard on the shoulders of *black* workers with *less than a high school diploma who were unemployed*; here we found that for the only year in which all workers answered the mastery questions, the same standout—low mastery—group emerged. Even more persuasively, the groups that were particularly low in depression—blacks and whites who had high school diplomas and were employed—were particularly high in mastery. For mastery, as was true of depression, black workers were especially sensitive to their level of educational attainment. In Chapter Five, we attributed the overall three–way linkage among race, education, and unemployment to the workers' assessments of their own human capital and their consequent visions of the future. Here we see that the linkage also holds in terms of the ability they feel they have to make that future.

Gender. The male–female difference in the impact of unemployment did not even approach significance. It also did not parallel Chapter Five's findings about gender and unemployment. Next we looked at men separately from women, controlling for other factors; we found that unemployment did not significantly affect mastery in men but did in women. (This is opposite to the pattern reported in Chapter Five, where unemployment significantly affected men's, but not women's, depression.) We explored whether or not the lack of significance in men resulted because some factor (such as financial hardship) more effectively accounted for unemployment's effects among men. We did find that when financial hardship and prior income were removed from our models, unemployment significantly decreased mastery among men. Even so, the relationship remained stronger among women.

One of the lessons to be learned from this pattern of mastery among men and women is that at least in this blue–collar sample, men's overall sense of mastery is closely tied to a complex of financial factors. The meaning of unemployment is financial, and unemployment's impact on mastery disappears when these financial factors are taken into account. Whatever work means to women, it appears to be empowering over and above its effect on their pocketbooks.

Gender, Mastery, Unemployment, and Depression. We next asked whether (1) unemployment and mastery interact in their effect on depression and (2) this effect differs between men and women. In statistical terms this last question refers to a three–way interaction: gender x unemployment x mastery. In regressions where other factors such as demographic characteristics were taken into account, this three–way interaction was not significant. Still, a two–way linkage emerged. Unemployment and mastery interacted significantly, such that unemployment increased depression less when people were high in mastery—and more, when they were low in mastery. Further, when we looked at men and women separately, we found no unemployment–mastery interaction at all for women, but a highly significant one for men. Gender specified the results, as Table 6.10 summarizes.

Chapter Five's results and the current ones, taken together, offer interesting food for thought about the meaning of jobs and job losses in these men and women. Seemingly, women feel the loss of a job in terms of a loss of mastery, and they do so to an even greater extent than men. Men's feeling that their mastery is slipping is linked closely to their financial status, but women's is not. Looking at depression, women feel more depressed than men, but their employment status has nothing much to do with it. Men's employment status is implicated in two ways: Unemployed men are significantly more depressed, and the impact of unemployment depends on a man's sense of mastery. It appears that for women, jobs have a meaning which is less clearly and simply financial (as the results for mastery indicate), and life can take on a grim quality that is hardly touched by getting a job (as the results for depression show).

Our data show clearly that to be worth less financially affects the sense of psychological worth. Being worth less is implicated in feeling worthless. Thus, for these workers, worth less can be equated to feeling worthless. This is one of the particularly pernicious effects of losing one's job.

Table 6.10

Predicting W1–W3 Change in Depression:
Gender Differences in the Role of Mastery and Unemployment
(Unstandardized Coefficients) [a]

	Men N = 803	Women 187
Mastery (M)	$-.17$	$^{c}-.27^{b}$
Unemployment (U)	$.81^{c}$	$-.03$
M x U	$-.22^{c}$	$-.01$
$R^{2} =$	$.53$	$.52$

[a] N = 990. All control variables from prior tables (race, age, etc.) were also included in these analyses.
[b] $p < .05$.
[c] $p < .01$.

SUMMING UP: WORTH AND WORTHLESSNESS

The first section of this chapter, which focuses on financial hardship, is intimately connected to the later sections dealing with the self. Together, financial hardship and self–constructs like mastery and self–esteem provide the two great paths between a crisis like job loss and consequences like personal distress or family conflict. Financial hardship (to be "worth less") generates distress directly, in and of itself; it also produces changes in views of the self (to feel worthless and powerless) which themselves contribute to distress. This linkage is intimate enough and inevitable enough that worthlessness and powerlessness are sometimes thought of as symptoms, not causes, of depression. Later, Chapter Eight illustrates some of the ways in which autoworkers caught up in a plant closing were able to avoid the equation of "worth less" with "worthless."

7

The Persistence of Stress: Negative Life Events in the Recent and Distant Past

Don't get me wrong, my home life wasn't always very good. When I worked, I wasn't around very much. I didn't think of myself as a big family man, but I did see myself as a work–every–day kind of provider. Then I wasn't a provider. I was suddenly home all the time with a marriage that was never any good to start with. At least work had kept me out of the house and the pay check kept things kind of even. Nothing about what I was seemed to be there anymore. I felt down all the time, but I was the kind of guy who got his mind off his problems by getting busy. When I was out and not sure I'd get back into GM, I was just in a fog, you know, I wasn't sure about anything. As time went on I found out what it means to be depressed. I don't think I'll ever tell anyone who's down to "snap out of it" anymore—that's not the way it is in reality.

—a closing plant worker

This chapter, like its predecessor, concerns those elements the person adds to the equation to convert stressful times into personal distress. This chapter addresses the way events in the immediate or distant past shaped responses to unemployment in our study. Each builds upon earlier chapters. Chapter Three laid out the overall dimensions of the unemployment that followed the 1987 GM plant closings and Chapter Four traced the patterns of individual and family distress. Just as Chapter Five concentrated on the roles and statuses to which identity is attached, Chapter Six concentrated on the self. Chapter Five pointed out that workers did not really talk about their identities in terms of race or gender. Similarly, except for the closing of the GM plants, they also tended to talk about ongoing conditions rather than events. For example, the quote earlier from a closing plant worker describes some of the way a bad situation is made worse when a blow like unemployment is coupled with previous or ongoing stress. The bad marriage referred to here is a chronic stressor; a separation or divorce, in contrast, is a stressful event. Both are important. The events are easier to ask about. Because chronic stressors also play a role in the stress process (Pearlin, 1989), it is important not to assume that the questions we asked tapped everything about workers' pasts that would be relevant to their stress responses to unemployment.

All too often, a previous or concurrent stressor worsens the situation either by simply adding up to "too much," when coupled with unemployment, or by sensitizing the worker to unemployment. The first of these, statistically speaking, is a main effect of the event; the second is an interactive effect in which the person who has experienced the prior stressor is more reactive (what is usually termed more vulnerable) to the later stressor. In this chapter, we have the unusual opportunity to explore two kinds of prior stressors:

1. For the entire sample of workers, each survey asked a standard checklist of items covering things that might have happened in the previous 12 months (described in Chapter Two); these kinds of checklists capture immediate, recent, and potentially ongoing sources of distress.

2. We asked the male workers about military experience; if the worker responded that he had such experience, we asked about combat; and if the worker had been in combat, we found out to which war he was referring. (None of the women in the sample reported having military experience.)

Although data about military experience are relevant only to the males in our sample (about 80%), it makes it possible to address the impact of a stressor—combat—about which much has been written. Combat experiences of these men involved different cohorts fighting different wars, as long as 40 or more years before we interviewed them.   The remainder of the chapter first offers a general overview of these two types of events, then reports on the impact of recent life stressors for the main sample, and finally goes into greater depth in discussing the role of prior combat in the experience of unemployment. The latter discussion draws on a paper by Calvin et al. (1996).

STRESS ACROSS THE LIFE COURSE

Chapter One outlined how our work draws on both the life course perspective and on stress research. From a life course perspective, the stress response depends upon what the individual brings to the experience. The person who reaches a life course transition with one set of experiences differs from the person with another set in ways that can shape their perceptions of the situation and the paths they subsequently follow. This means that although a person's response to a current stressor is a function of the social characteristics—such as race and gender—that were the focus of Chapter Five, it is not solely a function of these forces. Previous stressful events shape a person's later responses to stress (Elder, 1985, 1994; Moen, Kain, & Elder, 1983). A large volume of research documents that both discrete stressful events and chronic role strains are associated with poorer mental health, especially depression and anxiety (e.g., Pearlin, 1989; Thoits, 1995). This chapter focuses on the way sequential stressors string themselves together in the life course: when and how one stressful experience affects the person's ability to cope with a later experience. These are what Thoits (1995) calls "carryover" effects.

An earlier stressful event or condition—whether it occurred two months or twenty years earlier—can logically have two kinds of effects on distress. It can, in itself, cause distress for a number of reasons. Among these are the simple memory of the event (a spouse died), the changes in one's life that resulted from the event (the house had to be sold), or the behavioral changes that ensued (the survivor lost contact with neighbors and became lonely). In contrast, carryover effects mean that an *old* stressor affects the way a *new* stressor is reacted to, whether or not the old stressor in itself continues to create distress. Statistically, the continuing impact of an earlier stressor is a main effect; the impact on the way a new stressor is handled is an interactive effect. We will explore two kinds of prior stressful event/experience:

negative life events in the past year
military combat
for evidence of two kinds of effects:
a main effect (prior events generate distress)
an interaction (prior events increase distress in response to a current event).

Hundreds of studies in recent decades have been devoted to the potential health consequences of "negative life events"; these are sets of events that generally involve losses or threats of some sort, which create distress. They are stressful. In fact, the original research in this area by Holmes and Rahe (1967) assumed that change of any kind is stressful; they included checklists of positive things (marriage) as well as negative things (divorce) that could happen to change a person's life. Now it is generally agreed that positive life events have little effect on mental health. What matters is life's negatives (Thoits, 1983).

The next section of this chapter concentrates on a set of the standard "negative life events" (recent or concurrent stressful events) that are usually studied, showing what they are and how common they are. As noted before, this part of our investigation of negative life events involves *all workers*. Later in this chapter, when we turn from the immediate past to the influence of a long–ago stressor, we must restrict the sample because the stressor (combat) affects only *male workers*. Although this narrows the scope of the conclusions we can draw in one sense—we lose information about the way women carry along scars over time—it is clearly advantageous to study the impact of a serious stressor with long–term impacts. For each of these types of stressor, unemployment represents an additional "negative life event." Taken together, the two investigations help to paint a picture of the way the effects of stressors can accumulate at any given time and how they can resonate over the years.

NEGATIVE LIFE EVENTS IN THE IMMEDIATE PAST

The most important "negative life events" from a theoretical point of view are events that occur before unemployment happens (or, in a study like ours, before the announcement of plant closing). Only these events can confidently be described as occurring independently of the plant closing experience. In the following discussion we do not stop with the Wave 1 measures of prior stressful events, however. We also describe the frequency of stressful events reported and their apparent relationship to unemployment throughout the panel study, to get some picture of the way negative life experiences do or do not become interwoven with joblessness as causes of misery. In short, negative things that occur in lives can cause misery; but misery can also cause negative things to happen. A panel study like our own enables us to look at these negative life events in both ways.

Negative Life Events at the Outset of the Study

Table 7.1 reports three summaries of negative life events—primary events to the self, secondary events to the self, and overall events (including to spouse and children) as of Wave 1 of the survey. It shows how each of these measures relates to employment status, race, and gender. Where the relationship is significant, asterisk(s) appear beside the right–hand member of each pair of scores. For

Table 7.1
Primary, Secondary, and Overall Negative Life Events at Wave 1:
Sums of Events by Employment Status, Race, and Gender [a]

	Employed	Unemployed	White	Black	Male	Female
Primary	.87	.93	.84	1.01[b]	.81	1.17[b]
Secondary	.34	.32	.34	.31	.33	.36
Overall	1.06	1.14	1.04	1.17	1.03	1.24[b]

[a] Overall events includes primary and secondary events to the person, plus events to spouse and children. Cases were restricted to workers who responded at all waves and were either white or black (N = 1,047).
[b] Significantly different from the sum to its immediate left at p < .05.

consistency across waves and across chapters of this book, the analysis is restricted to workers who had data at all three surveys, were either white or black, and were not retired by Wave 2 or 3 of the study.

Significant results are sparse. Employment status is unrelated to any measure of negative life events. This means that we are in the enviable position—statistically at least—of studying what happens when a person's life woes are increased by a genuinely unrelated, separate source of stress (unemployment). Race, in contrast, shows some relationship to the experience of negative life events; blacks are significantly more likely than whites to report primary life events (but not secondary events or overall number of events). Gender shows more differentiation still; women report more primary life events and more overall events than men. It is necessary to ask, however, whether this gender difference is real. Recall that women were asked about a few events—like miscarriage—that could not occur to men. Thus we could expect that their report of primary life events might be inflated. This can be assessed by examining gender differences in the score for overall life events. The overall score incorporates into the totals for the married men (who form the bulk of the male sample) those same female–specific items like miscarriage, which they are asked about as "negative events to the spouse." Gender differences exist for both primary events and overall events, suggesting that there was a genuine difference between men and women and that women reported experiencing more negative events during the year before our first interview with them.

In all waves of the study, females reported significantly more nonfinancial negative life events than males, just as blacks reported more than whites. In contrast to the findings for overall negative life events and for primary life events, events to others did not differentiate men and women. Men and women looked more similar than different in their reactions to negative life events which occurred to their spouse (effect minimal for both) or to their children (effect sizeable for both).

Trends in Negative Life Events

Although our main theoretical interest in negative life events lies in their ability to predispose a person to be susceptible to a new stressor and hence to act as an independent variable in the stress equation, it is valuable to ask what happens to the pattern of negative life events over time. Negative life events can be an interesting dependent variable in their own right. For example, we have already noted that it is predictable (almost tautological) if the secondary life events that normally accompany a financial crisis increase after unemployment. It is more interesting if, for example, ties with loved ones more often break following unemployment (see Chapter Four). And finally, what is an effect at one point can become a cause at another: Whatever happens to negative life events, they presumably affect a worker's distress at later points—such as the next wave of our survey.

Our analysis for each of the four types of negative events crosses the three waves of the survey: the three categories of primary events, plus secondary events. We compared closing and nonclosing plant workers rather than the unemployed versus the employed to make consistent comparisons across the entire study. A worker's initial closing/nonclosing plant placement is constant over time, whereas employment status shifts from wave to wave. The analysis used adjusted scores (using an analysis of covariance)for both closing and nonclosing plant workers, taking into account the fact that these groups differed on a number of important personal characteristics (see Chapter Two). For example, because nonclosing plant workers were older than closing plant workers and more often married, more of them could be expected to have spouses die simply for these reasons.

This analysis (not shown) offers insights about the overall incidence of negative life events, about initial closing/nonclosing plant differences in their frequency, and about the differential toll taken over time in each group of workers:

First, overall incidence. First and foremost, negative life events of all kinds are rare, as evidenced by the low sums for events of every type. Although some workers may have experienced more than one of life's crises and tragedies, it is unlikely that these numbers could be so small unless most workers escaped tragedy altogether. Second, group differences. Closing plant workers looked no different from their counterparts in nonclosing plants on some measures at Wave 1. Of more interest to us, by and large they showed the same patterns of change and stability over time as the nonclosing plant workers in some cases. For example, closing and nonclosing plant workers did not differ significantly with regard to trends in loss of loved ones. More importantly, they did not differ with regard to trends in primary life events as a whole, not between Wave 1 and Wave 2 and not between Wave 2 and Wave 3. Third, important trends. Workers from both groups collected additional negative events over time, but the largest toll of such events came for *closing plant workers* and involved the *secondary events*. The (upward) trend in secondary life events between Wave 1 and Wave 2 was highly significant in closing plants, but only marginally so in nonclosing plants (p = .07). Between Wave 2 and Wave 3, secondary events increased significantly only for closing plant workers. In other words, *one effect of the plant closing experience on workers was the fact that it led them to experience other (secondary) negative events.* The small and transient increase in secondary events for nonclosing plant workers between the first and second waves seems counterintuitive at first. Why should workers, who for the most part have *kept* their jobs, be reporting an increase in the largely financial secondary life events? Even though their tendency to report increased secondary events is weak, it seems to contradict these workers' relative financial position. We believe that the trend is real and that it can be understood in the context of genuine hardships that workers in the nonclosing plants were feeling. Preceding chapters showed that although most workers in nonclosing plants held onto their jobs, they generally saw their incomes stagnate and may even have experienced income losses because of loss of overtime. These workers also feared that their own jobs were in danger, as their elevated anxiety at Wave 1 showed. Either because of their experience of income squeeze or their fears of what was to come, this reaction makes sense. The kind of unemployment that rolls through a community when plants close is contagious. It is the kind of unemployment about which it is very easy for people to feel "I am next."

Of course, this analysis focuses on negative life events *per se*, rather than the distress that can be caused by those events. The linkage between these events and workers' distress is the subject of the next section.

Mental Health Effects of Negative Life Events

Main Effects. How much of a role do negative life events play in tearing further at the fabric of workers' daily lives and mental health? *First, in their own right they are a powerful determinant of depression.* (Similar results, not shown here, hold for anxiety, albeit more weakly, and for somatic symptoms and hostility, more weakly still. As in other chapters, we concentrate on depression because of its importance to mental health and its demonstrated lingering impact on the unemployed.)

Table 7.2 shows effects of primary and secondary life events on depression, controlled for workers' demographic characteristics, employment status, and financial hardships. The equations omit self–esteem and mastery because these cannot be studied across all three waves (see Chapter Six). In this table, results are presented in terms of unstandardized regression coefficients. This means that we can tell directly the size of the impact that a change of one unit in the predictor has on the predicted (depression). Because they are scaled the same, primary and secondary life events can be directly compared and/or added together into an estimate of the overall impact of negative events on the self. (Recall that this sum excludes negative events to spouse and children, so that the overall number of negative life events as a whole and their impact could be larger than appears here.)

Table 7.2 reveals differences between the types of negative events, as well as differences in potency between negative life events and the other factors studied. The table makes it clear that primary negative life events are strongly associated with depression. Equally clearly, the role of secondary events is minor and insignificant. (The latter result partially reflects the presence of financial hardship as a variable in the equation because secondary events are largely financial. Other analyses, not shown, revealed that the impact of secondary events was small even with financial hardship omitted.)

At each wave of the survey, negative life events (whether primary, or primary plus secondary) have *as big an impact* on depression as any single personal characteristic. Sometimes the effect is bigger. Only gender and race affect

Table 7.2
Effect of Negative Life Events on Depression Across the Panel Study [a]

	Wave 1	Wave 2	Wave 3
Control variables			
Race (1=black)	−.11[c]	−.14[c]	−.11[c]
Gender (1=female)	.16[c]	.09[c]	.08[b]
Married (1=yes)	−.03	−.06	−.04
Age	.03	.06[b]	.05
Education	:00	−.05	−.02
Income	.01	−.02	−.05
Life events			
Unemployed (1=yes)	.01	.02	.06
Primary events	.12[c]	.12[c]	.24[c]
Secondary events	.01	.05	.02
Related strains			
Financial hardship	.36[c]	.33[c]	.30[c]
$R^2 =$	.20	.20	.24

N = 996.
[b] $p < .05$.
[c] $p < .01$.

depression to a comparable extent, and the effects of both gender and race are more complex—interactive—than shown here (see Chapter Five). To sum up, the straightforward, simple, main effect of negative life events outweighs that of the standard sociological predictors. In fact, the impact of negative life events is dwarfed only by that of financial hardship; Chapter Six addressed the latter variable in greater detail. For present purposes, it is noteworthy that some financial items have a subjective cast (what is "not enough food"?), whereas negative life events at least appear more objective (a person dies, a house burns down). This means that the strong relationship between financial hardship and depression in our study and those of others may be more ambiguous than it is usually portrayed. Just as a financially strapped person is depressed, a depressed person may feel more financially strapped. Seen in that light, the results here probably inflate the impact of financial hardship relative to the impact of negative life events. In any case, primary negative life events emerge as a potent determinant of depression whose impact rivals or exceeds that of such traditional predictors as gender and race.

There is an applied or clinical side to these findings. Considering that many of the workers who spoke to us during the panel study experienced unemployment at some point and that unemployment itself is a potent negative life event, this means that numerous workers experienced two or more negative life events in any given year. When three or more negative events happen to a person in close proximity, clinically significant depression becomes highly likely (Brown & Harris, 1978; Monroe & Simons, 1991). The unemployed worker who experienced any one additional negative event was facing at least a two–strike count.

To sum up the basic relationship between negative life events and distress, especially depression, the first thing we expected to find—that negative life events are harmful to mental health—was true.

Interaction with Unemployment. The second thing we expected to find was that experiencing other negative life events would make people more vulnerable to the mental health impact of unemployment. We tested this through statistical interactions like those involving race, education, and unemployment in Chapter Five. We explored the potential interactive effect in various ways. First, all tests were carried out for both depression and anxiety and always for (a) primary and secondary events separately and (b) combined. Tests included (1) Considering the impact of cumulative unemployment as of Wave 3 and testing the life events–unemployment interaction by using as predictors the negative life events reported in Wave 3 that occurred in the previous year; (2) using as predictors a cumulative measure of all the negative life events of the entire study; and (3) taking unemployment at either Wave 1 or Wave 2 or Wave 3 separately, in combination with that wave's negative life events.

Table 7.3 summarizes what we found. For brevity, effects are reported only for unemployment, negative life events, and their interaction, although we always controlled for workers' demographic characteristics. To provide the most inclusive indicator of negative life events and to simplify the number of interactions estimated, we used the overall sum of negative life events (primary, secondary, to spouse, and to children). Coefficients for negative life events may differ from the coefficients already shown in Table 7.2 for a couple of reasons: A different life events measure is being used in Table 7.3, and the interaction term (unemployment x negative life events) is included in the equations.

Table 7.3 reveals *almost no evidence that negative life events make workers more vulnerable to the impact of unemployment.* Only at Wave 1 do we find any indications that this is so, and only for anxiety.

Overall, these patterns of difference and of movement over time suggest the following conclusions, at least for this study of workers subjected to plant closing: (1) Primary life events do not increase over time, whereas secondary events do. (2) Secondary life events do not affect mental health significantly, whereas primary events do. (3) Although the negative life events studied here have a powerful impact on workers' distress, prior negative events do not seem to make the worker's response to the later stressor, unemployment, any more severe.

These findings do *not* support an argument that life's crises build, cascade, or act upon one another to wear away the mental health of individuals. Yet the life course approach reviewed in Chapter One strongly suggests that what goes wrong at one life point should affect whether things go right or wrong down the road. What kind of thing should a researcher study to investigate this possibility? Optimally, research on stress in the life course should address events or life transitions that are clearly definable, deemed important in the culture, and widely shared. It may be that research that draws on traditional life events research is overly restricted, in particular by the emphasis on both recent and discrete happenings in the checklists, such as were used here. After all, the life course approach was forged during studies of "events" such as the Great Depression Elder, 1974) and World War II (Stouffer, Suchman, DeVinney, Star, & Williams, 1949). Especially for men, the potentially stressful experiences of military service and unemployment have been clearly definable, important, and commonplace. To explore these issues, we look next at the impact of a powerful, but in this case, long–ago stressor, men's experiences of combat during war. Although this restricts the size of the sample and the generalizability of the results, it focuses on a stressor that may be particularly powerful in the blue–collar group of men we studied.

Table 7.3

Effects of Negative Life Events, Unemployment, and their Interactions on Depression, Anxiety, and Hostility Across the Panel Study [a]

| | Wave 1 | | |
	Depression	Anxiety	Hostility
Negative life events (NLE).	13[c]	.08[b]	.11[c]
Unemployment (U)	.01	−.00	.03
NLE x U	.01	.08[b]	−.03
R^2 =	.20	.15	.19

| | Wave 2 | | |
	Depression	Anxiety	Hostility
Negative life events (NLE).	.15	.09[b]	.12[c]
Unemployment (U)	.02	.01	.05
NLE x U	-.01	.06	−.07
R^2 =	.20	.15	.13

| | Wave 3 | | |
	Depression	Anxiety	Hostility
Negative life events (NLE).	.27[c]	.17[b]	.19[c]
Unemployment (U)	.05	.06	.05
NLE x U	.00	-.02	−.08
R^2 =	.24	.13	.14

[a] N ranged from 981 to 988. Equations controlled for race, gender, marital status, years of education, age, prior income, and financial hardship during the previous year. Without financial hardship in the model, unemployment was always a significant predictor of depression and anxiety; see the following discussion of combat as a stressor.
[b] $p < .05$.
[c] $p < .01$.

CARRYOVER EFFECTS OF A PRIOR STRESSOR

Mechanisms of Carryover

Some explanations of carryover phenomena stress discontinuities; others, continuities. We might think of three broad categories of mechanisms that may underlie the persistence of stress symptoms (Elder, 1985; 1994; Moen et al., 1983; Thoits, 1995):

1. *Interactional continuity.* A person's pattern of behavior toward others tends to recreate the same (stress–provoking) conditions over and over again. For example, hostility tends to evoke responses that maintain hostility.

2. *Cumulative effects.* Behavioral continuity can be maintained through a progressive accumulation of the consequences of the behavior itself (Elder, 1985; 1994). For example, hostility can threaten a marriage or employment, consequences which themselves are stress–producing.

These first two processes are sources of continuity between an earlier stress and a later self. They are likely to be interrelated. When an early stressor generates maladaptive behavior such as hostility, the first of these processes says that the hostility is likely to be maintained over time via social interaction. The second process says that it is likely to be exacerbated by the unfortunate consequences that follow on such behavior.

3. *Situational activation.* New events and new stressors can also serve as reminders of the old based on their similarity (usually a similarity in loss of control). This process is more discontinuous; a person is reminded anew of something *from the past.*

This notion is similar to a state of hypervigilance: people who have experienced a trauma such as combat may be more likely to notice, to pick out, the negative and stressful aspects of a new situation. They may react to more situations, and/or react more extremely to a given situation, than those who were not traumatized. To the extent that the person is hypervigilant, the process of situational activation becomes more continuous; the continuity simply involves perceptions rather than behaviors.

Identity. In the United States, "Enlisted service was the modal experience for young American men from the eve of World War II until the end of the draft following the Vietnam War" (Moskos, 1986, p. 35). When the economic disruption we were studying began (1987), it was estimated that more than one–third of all adult males in this country served in the military. Indeed, for most of this century, "being a man" in America has traditionally meant being willing to fight for one's homeland, to work for a living, and to support a family in wedlock (Brod, 1992; Farrell, 1993; Kimmel, 1996; Ross & Huber, 1985). The salient role–identities (see Stryker, 1980; Thoits, 1991) can be described as those of *warrior, worker (producer)*, and *provider.* Here we attempt to discover what effects, if any, the warrior role had on a man's reaction to disruption of the worker role later on.

Cohorts and the Life Course

The individual moves through social life in a dimension of place (locations and roles) and a dimension of time (the era or period, on the one hand, and the phase of the person's life cycle, on another). With regard to time, all events occur at an intersection. The person stands in a particular period in history, at a particular point in the life cycle. In social science, this intersection is captured by in the concept of the cohort, individuals who encounter a given historical event or change at the same stage in their life cycles (Ryder, 1965). In statistical terms, a cohort is the interaction of (historical) period and (personal) age or seniority. Differences in the nature of the events to which people are exposed during military service may have profound implications for the later life cycle.

The question is how to look for cohort effects in the arena of military service. First, it is vital to pull apart the institutional effects of military service, the contextual effects of wartime versus peacetime service, and the personal impact of combat. Doing so is easiest if a researcher can identify and study multiple periods of alternating experiences. Logically, the "war" (A) and "peace" (nonwar) (B) periods of recent U.S. history form an A–B–A–B design. As applied to people still active in the labor force at the time of our surveys, this design has at least six elements (periods): World War II, the interwar before Korea, Korea, the interwar before Vietnam, Vietnam, and post–Vietnam. (For data sets that extend into the 1990s, the Gulf War and its aftermath could be added to this sequence.) To study combat experiences in two wars separated by an historical gap makes it easier to rule out some explanations (e.g., historical period) for any findings.

War Cohorts. Evidence about the impact of military service on men's mental health is mixed. Elder and his colleagues studied the impact of military experience during the World War II and Korean eras on the Terman cohort (born 1903–1920), the Oakland cohort (born 1920–1921), and the Berkeley cohort (born 1928–1929) (Elder, Gimbel, & Ivie, 1991). This research indicated that military service *per se* could represent a "time out" and a "turning point" in careers, with generally beneficial consequences (Elder, 1986; Elder & Hareven, 1993). In contrast, studies of Vietnam veterans have tended to show negative effects (e.g., Boulanger & Kadushin, 1986; Card, 1983; Frey–Wouters & Laufer, 1986). The most thorough investigation with a nonclinical sample is probably that by Vinokur, Caplan, & Williams (1987), who studied men born largely in the post–World War II period, from the 1940s to mid–1950s, early in the "baby boom." The psychological effects of both military service during the era and combat in Vietnam were negative.

In neither the research program by Elder nor the Vinokur et al. (1987) study is a clear distinction drawn among the institutional effects of military service *per se*, the social context of military service during wartime versus peace, the experiential effects of combat, and the differences that may emerge as a function of a particular war. The military service variable for Elder's Berkeley sample combines the last two years of World War II, the Korean war, and the peacetime years in between (e.g., Elder, 1986). Thus, Elder does not distinguish between the effects of military service during wartime and service during peace. Vinokur et al. (1987) contrast those who served in Vietnam, those who served outside the war theater, and nonveterans who were eligible for service during the same period; their time frame was entirely wartime. For different reasons, then, Vinokur et al. also cannot tease out the impact of military service *per se* from its wartime or peacetime social context. We were able to tease out and test most of these potential differences.

What We Expected to Find

In this case, the long–ago stressor was combat, and its context was military experience; the current stressor was joblessness and the attendant financial hardship. To provide further context, we also took account not only of the worker's marital status and also of whether his wife was working. We will explain our choices later.

Military Service. Military service *per se* has generally positive and long–lasting effects. This is true for a number of reasons—the ways in which the military serves as a beneficial "time out" in the male's life span, the training and resources it provides, and the benefits (e.g., comradeship; Elder & Clipp, 1988a, b) it continues to make available to the veteran in later life. Combat, in contrast, is associated with distress (e.g., Helzer, Robins, & Davis, 1976; Segal, 1977; U.S./CDC, 1988). We expected to find that combat veterans experience greater anxiety, depression, and/or hostility and that this effect of combat might be particularly pronounced for anxiety symptoms, given that posttraumatic stress disorder (PTSD) is an anxiety disorder. In addition to combat's direct negative influence on mental health, we also looked for a *carryover* effect. If carryover occurs, combat predisposes its veterans to be more vulnerable to the negative mental health impacts of joblessness and the financial hardship that accompanies it.

The effects of *joblessness* and *financial hardship* have been encountered throughout this book. Either or both of these conditions is associated with distress, especially with depression and anxiety. In contrast, marriage is typically associated with lower rates of depression among men. A marriage partner provides social support which is known to improve mental health directly and to aid in coping with stressors, including job loss (e.g., Kessler et al., 1985). Given these benefits of marriage, married men should be at an advantage, relative to the unmarried, in coping with a stressor like combat: Combat should have a bigger effect on distress among the unmarried (see Elder & Clipp, 1988a, b, 1989; Ivie, Gimbel, & Elder, 1991; Thoits, 1995).

The possible role of spousal employment is less clear, and we include it on an exploratory basis only because it may give us further insight into these men's understanding of the provider role. Economically speaking, a working wife enlarges the family income, which relieves financial hardship, and is generally found to alleviate men's distress (Pearlin et al., 1981). But there is also an more emotional meaning to whether or not a wife works. Research shows that in couples with traditional sex role attitudes and men with unstable work histories, a working wife increases the husband's distress. Presumably, this is due to the threat to the husband's provider role (Ross, Mirowsky, & Huber, 1983). The impact of spousal employment can also vary across classes and cohorts (Campbell, 1984; Wandersee–Bolin, 1978, Wandersee, 1981). Working class and older individuals each are more likely to take traditional sex role attitudes.

We did not expect to see an effect of spousal employment in these panel data, because the financially related positive impact of a wife's employment could be counteracted by its psychological costs in a population likely to hold relatively traditional sex role attitudes.

Cohorts. There are a number of reasons to expect mental health differences between cohorts, especially between men eligible for military service during World War II/Korea and those eligible during Vietnam:

1. Wars differ. World War II at one extreme and Vietnam at the other differed in the level of support from the citizenry, in the conventional versus guerrilla nature of the conflict, and in the aftermaths to which veterans returned. Many studies have documented the positive reception of returning veterans after World War II and the negative responses of the American public to the Vietnam war and other wars (Figley & Leventman, 1980; Severo & Milford, 1989).

2. Whether or not veterans were in combat, they returned to quite different labor markets at different points in history. The "Children of the Great Depression" studied by Elder (1974) experienced their period of key career and family formation years (ages 25–44) after World War II and Korea, but before 1973. Conversely, since 1973, several factors have put pressures on American men's identity as provider. Real wages stagnated between 1973 and 1986. Moreover, although the wages of both college– and high school–educated young men declined after 1973, those of the less educated were more affected and the gap between them grew (Levy, 1987; Levy & Michel, 1991).

Thus, Vietnam veterans—who were, after all, the grandchildren of the Great Depression—experienced a rockier transition to and progression through civilian careers after wartime than was true of their parents' generation.

Research Methods

Variables Unique to these Analyses. Most of the variables under study here are the same as throughout the rest of the book, but a few are unique to the investigation of the role of combat, and others are defined or used somewhat differently from other chapters. Following we briefly summarize the way new variables were conceptualized and how certain familiar variables were looked at differently: Military service *per se* was a dummy variable (0 = never served/ 1 = ever served). Military cohort and combat status were derived from the preceding item in combination with follow–up questions. Workers who had served in the military were asked (a) whether this was during a war (and if so which one) and (b) whether they served in combat. Combat is a dummy variable (0=no, with or without military service; 1=yes). To make the best use of the sometimes limited numbers of older veterans, we defined *military cohorts* as consisting of four periods, that is, we combine World War II and Korea into a single war cohort and two interwar periods, 1946–1949 and 1953–1963, into a single nonwar cohort. The result is a somewhat condensed A–B–A–B (war/peace, war/peace) design: (1) a World War II/Korea cohort; (2) the interwar periods (1946–1949, 1953–1963); (3) Vietnam; and (4) the post–Vietnam period. We constructed four dummy variables, where 1 = served during World War II or Korea; 1 = served in an interwar period between World War II and Korea or between Korea and Vietnam; 1 = served during Vietnam; 1 = served in the post–Vietnam period. In each case, 0 = was of the same age range but did not serve. This cohort definition has the advantage of providing a large enough N in each cohort to allow for multivariate analyses and allows us to test for a peacetime–wartime distinction. Its costs include the fact that it groups together two different wars, World War II and Korea, and that its "interwar" period is not continuous but consists of two distinct time periods, 1946–49 and 1953–63. Any person who served in the military across more than one period was coded in accordance with two rules: (a) assign to the earlier period, unless (b) the man has earlier peacetime service, followed by combat—in which case, assign to the wartime period in which combat occurred.

Joblessness (1 = employed/ 0 = not employed) was defined less restrictively than in other analyses, so that the "not employed" group included a small number of retirees, as well as workers who voluntarily remained out of the labor force (Hamilton et al., 1993). To the extent that these latter groups are less mentally distressed than the involuntarily unemployed, employment status as defined here may underestimate the distress of the jobless, but it serves the important function of retaining cases for cohort analyses.

Spousal employment was a dummy variable (employed spouse = 1; all others = 0). All other variables and demographic controls were measured as in previous chapters. As in the earlier part of this chapter, age rather than seniority is included among the controls because it is more directly relevant to the current emphasis on the life course. In keeping with the results reported earlier in this chapter, analyses also controlled for other negative life events experienced during the previous year. *Models To Be Tested.* We were concerned with four basic issues: (1) the condition of the workers at the start of the study, Wave 1; (2) how they fared from Wave 1 to Wave 3 (their change in distress); (3) how combat affected distress or change in distress; and (4) how cohorts differed. The next section presents the results of our tests for each of these issues, looking at three dependent variables, depression, anxiety, and hostility.

The basic regression model for each dependent variable includes the independent variables military service, combat, employment status, marital status, and spousal employment. In assessing baseline distress, we used Wave 1 measures of all variables. In assessing change in distress by Wave 3, Wave 3 marital status is used so as to capture important changes (marriages, divorces) that might contribute to men's distress.

Controls always include age, race, education, income, and negative life events (other than joblessness). Regressions that tested for cohort differences replaced military service with dummies for military cohort (served=1, did not serve = 0). When both military service (or military cohort dummies) and combat status are included in a regression, the coefficient for military service (or for military cohorts) can be read as the effect of military service without experiencing combat. In models with military cohort dummies, age effects refer to age variation within the cohort. Multivariate analyses are restricted to those who responded at all waves of the survey and had complete data on the dependent variables, independent variables, and controls. Following, we present results first for Wave 1 distress and then for change scores (Wave 3, controlling for Wave 1), in the same order.

Baseline Model

The left side of Table 7.4 presents the Wave 1 (baseline) effects of *war* (military service and combat); *work* (employment status and financial hardship), and *wedlock* (marital status and spousal employment), in order. Change over time (Wave 1–Wave 3) appears on the right.

The effects of the war–related variables were essentially nil at the start of our study. Military service does not benefit and combat does not harm mental health, as shown on the left side of Table 7.4. However, workers already knew at this point that plants would be closing, and some were already losing jobs. It is possible that the residual effects of a long–ago stressor, even a relatively potent one such as combat, were overwhelmed by the anxiety–provoking aspects of the current economic situation under these circumstances.

The impact of work versus joblessness was as expected. Financial hardship is a highly significant predictor of depression, anxiety, and hostility. The impact of joblessness on anxiety is significant, even controlling for hardship; jobless workers were more anxious than those who had jobs. (As in the first half of the chapter, initial analyses which included joblessness without financial hardship showed that job loss increased all three forms of distress.) Results are consistent with the argument that financial hardship largely—but not entirely—accounts for the impact of job loss on mental health.

At Wave 1, married workers were also less depressed. Although having a working wife was associated with somewhat higher depression and hostility, no effects of spousal employment reached significance.

Table 7.4

Impacts of Military Service, Employment, and Marital Status on Symptoms of Depression, Anxiety, and Hostility [a]

	Depression	Wave 1 Anxiety	Hostility	Wave 1 – Wave 3 Change Depression	Anxiety	Hostility
Intercept						
b	1.12^c	1.28^c	1.42^c	$.85^c$	$.91^c$	$.87^c$
War						
Military (M)						
b	−.05	.01	.02	−.06	−.17	−.03
Combat c						
b	.03	−.00	.02	.06	$.30^b$	$.11^b$
Work						
Employment (E)						
b	−.02	$−.12^b$	−.06	−.07	−.05	.02
Financial hardship (F)						
b	$.008^c$	$.005^c$	$.006^c$	$.004^c$	$.002^c$	$.004^c$
Military x F						
b				−.001		
Combat x F						
b					$.004^b$	
Wedlock						
Marital Status (MS)						
b	$−.14^b$	−.09	−.05	$−.11^c$	−.05	−.02
Spouse works (SP.W)						
b	.06	.00	.07	.04	.02	.06
Military x MS						
b				.14		
Combat x MS						
b					$−.36^c$	
Wave 1 distress						
b				$.37^c$	$.36^c$	$.30^c$
$R^2 =$	.19	.12	.13	.39	.28	.27

[a] N = 852 complete cases at Wave 1 and 864 cases at Wave 3. Controls include race, age, education, prior income, and other negative life events. Where preliminary analyses showed that interactions of combat or military experience with other variables were insignificant, models were reestimated deleting those terms (blanks above). When an interaction (e.g., combat x marital status) was significant, it was necessary for models to include its paired term (e.g., military x marital status), so that the significant coefficient would be interpretable. Wave 1 distress is included among the regressors only in the regressions on the right side of the table.
[b] p < .05.
[c] p < .01.

Change over Time

The right side of Table 7.4 shows trends over time between Wave 1 and Wave 3. Military service *per se* tended to *decrease* depression and anxiety over time, but combat significantly increased distress. Among combat veterans, anxiety and hostility were more likely to worsen—or fail to improve—over time. There was little change in depression. We have already suggested that the subtle impact of experiences like combat may have been washed out at Wave 1 by other stressors. Indeed, combat's role emerges over time in such phenomena as a persistently elevated level of anxiety. Table 7.4 shows that trends in distress over the two–year period of large–scale plant closings varied in response to aspects of military experiences that occurred decades earlier. These results for combat represent carryover effects of a prior stressor that are both long–term and highly meaningful for that substantial proportion of the population with military service.

Looking at change in distress offers a picture similar to Wave 1 distress in several cases. Financial hardship is consistently associated with more distress, whether the time frame is Wave 1 or Wave 1–Wave 3 change, and whether the distress is depression, anxiety, or hostility. Joblessness affects trends in depression over and above what is accounted for by financial hardship. Married respondents are less depressed than their unmarried counterparts. And there remains no significant impact of spousal employment. (In both cases, having an employed spouse is associated with greater distress, but the results are not significant.)

Combat and Carryover Stress

We originally expected that joblessness, financial hardship, or both might worsen distress to a greater extent for those men who were combat veterans (a carryover effect). The right side of Table 7.4 shows that this pattern occurs for change in distress over time: Combat and financial hardship interacted, meaning that hardships increased anxiety to a greater extent in combat veterans. When we looked at joblessness instead of financial hardship, the same patterns emerged but more weakly (and only for anxiety).

Combat and Marital Status in Combination. The right side of Table 7.4 also shows a significant interaction between combat and marital status with a change in anxiety. Among married men, neither military service nor combat had an effect on anxiety. But among the unmarried, anxiety was (a) worse for those with no military experience than for those who served in the military (but not in combat) and (b) worst of all for unmarried combat veterans. This result is consistent with Elder and Clipp's (1988a, b) finding that it was important to have a wife or friend with whom to share and relive combat experiences. Of course, these results are correlational and do not establish causation. It is possible, for example, that men who are highly anxious—perhaps as a result of combat—tend not to be selected or retained as marriage partners.

Cohort Differences. Cohort differences at Wave 1 of the study were not of interest, because Table 7.4 has already shown that military experience and combat had no effects on distress at that point.

Table 7.5 shows how the military cohorts differed concerning change in distress from Wave 1 to Wave 3. The results of Table 7.5 are drawn from regressions in which three military cohort dummies were included in each equation to replace the military service variable. (Post–Vietnam was the excluded category to which the other categories were compared.) For brevity, this table presents only the coefficients for the military cohort dummies and for combat, and leaves out the various controls that were included in the analysis; results for these variables not depicted were essentially the same as in the right side of Table 7.4.

The first three rows of Table 7.5 show the impact of serving in the military without experiencing combat in each of three periods—World War II/Korea, interwar, and Vietnam—relative to the post–Vietnam period. The fourth row shows the impact of combat *per se.* Coefficients for World War II/Korea and Vietnam military service are similar in sign and size; they tend to be significant only for the Vietnam cohort simply because there were many more Vietnam veterans. In general, a veteran who served in wartime (but not in combat) is less anxious than either those who did not serve at all or those who lived through combat. In contrast, combat veterans are more anxious, more hostile, and somewhat more depressed than all others.

Despite the suggestions reviewed earlier that Vietnam veterans might fare worse than their World War II/Korea counterparts, on the whole, we found no differences between the two wartime cohorts themselves. Table 7.5 showed that membership in the two military cohorts (without combat) had quite similar and positive effects. We also directly compared the effects of combat for military veterans in these wartime cohorts by creating a dummy variable (0 = World War II/Korea, 1 = Vietnam) and analyzed the differences between the wars, between combat and its absence among veterans, and the interaction between these wars and combat. Exploratory analyses of covariance for each form of distress, restricted to those with military service, showed no significant interactions. Combat in Vietnam had no greater, or smaller, effect on levels of distress than combat during World War II/Korea.

A more finely–tuned look provides some evidence, however, that Vietnam veterans may be more vulnerable to later stressors such as unemployment.

Table 7.5
Cohort and Combat Effects on Change in Mental Health (Wave 1 to Wave 3) [a]

	Depression	Anxiety	Hostility
World War II/Korea	−.08	−.09	−.03
Interwar	−.02	−.01	.01
Vietnam	−.07	−.10[b]	−.04
Combat	.08	.16[c]	.13[b]

[a] N = 864. Models replaced the military service term with three dummies for the historical periods in which men served or were eligible for service; the excluded category is post–Vietnam. As in Table 1, we included controls (race, age, education, prior income, and negative life events), employment status, marital status, spousal employment, combat experience, financial hardship, and the Wave 1 measure of each type of distress (turning the dependent variable into a change score). Effects not shown were substantively the same as earlier.
[b] $p < .05$.
[c] $p < .01$.

Table 7.6 shows the result of an exploratory breakdown of the World War II/Korea versus Vietnam cohorts. We focus on unmarried men, a high–risk group. (Note that the table's means are not adjusted for covariates such as race, education, or income because of the small number of World War II/Korea veterans).

In each column, we can directly compare results for each measure of distress as reported by the Vietnam veterans versus the World War II/Korea veterans. Here we make statistical comparisons as a descriptive tool. We concentrate first where we would expect the maximum impact of war, the unmarried combat veterans. The unmarried Vietnam veteran, much more so than his World War II/Korea counterpart, reports being severely depressed, anxious, and hostile. The effect for depression and hostility was significant, and that for anxiety was marginally so. Overall, *Vietnam combat veterans who were unmarried* had worse mental health than any other group. Cohort differences in the rest of the table are more subtle, and generally involve an advantage for the World War II/Korea cohort. This means that Table 7.6 is consistent with many popular and social scientific writings about the differences between World War II/Korea veterans and their Vietnam counterparts.

What Can We Conclude?

Negative life events, as they are most often studied by social scientists, were both important and relatively uninteresting in this case. Descriptively, it is important to know that a tally of the negative things that happen to a person predicts that person's levels of distress, and the results reconfirmed this notion. But negative life events of the recent past, captured by popular checklists, were rather statistically "inert." They did not carryover, that is, change the person's way of facing the next negative life event.

What we were looking for, and what the life course approach has taken as an assumption, is an interconnectedness among life's happenings, a sense that a biography is a meticulously constructed building rather than an inflatable tent. Carryover effects—in which experiencing one stressor changes the person's way of facing another—are part of this building process.

Military service without the experience of combat was associated with men reporting fewer symptoms of distress in this study (consistent with the results of Elder, 1986; Elder & Hareven, 1993; and Elder et al., 1991). On the other hand, military service with combat was harmful (consistent with such studies as Vinokur et al., 1987). Putting the two together, we found that noncombat veterans had the

Table 7.6

Wave 3 Mental Health of Unmarried Men:
World War II/Korea Versus Vietnam Cohorts [a]

	No Military Service	Military, No Combat	Military, Combat
Depression [b]			
World War II/Korea			
M	1.28	1.57	1.25
SD	.34	.42	.25
Vietnam			
M	1.58	1.53	1.94
SD	.54	.39	.97
Anxiety [b]			
World War II/Korea			
M	1.40	1.29	1.37
SD	.59	.28	.34
Vietnam			
M	1.34	1.20	1.72
SD	.50	.24	.91
Hostility [b]			
World War II/Korea			
M	1.25	1.39	1.13
SD	.46	.40	.21
Vietnam			
M	1.60	1.37	1.78
SD	.64	.31	.88

[a] Raw means were not adjusted for covariates because of small and uneven cell sizes. World War II/Korea N's = 15 (unmarried men with no military service), 9 (service, no combat), and 6 (combat); Vietnam N's were 52, 15, and 18.
[b] World War II/Korea vs. Vietnam combat veterans: Depression, post hoc t = 2.85, p = .0045; Anxiety, t = 1.67, p = .09; Hostility, t = 2.62, p = .009.

least distress of all. Such results offer a note of caution for those who do research on the impact of Vietnam or any other war. To examine "veterans" by combining combat veterans with veterans who did not experience combat is a mistake. It potentially lumps together those who were hurt and those who were helped by serving in the military. It can even yield an apparent absence of impact instead of the two opposite impacts that occurred.

Combat also interacted with financial hardship and formed a classic carryover effect. Combat veterans reacted to financial hardship with an increase in anxiety to a greater extent than those who did not see combat.

Wars differed, although it is difficult to be sure why. Detailed inspection of the wartime cohorts revealed a concentration of high–distress men who were unmarried, Vietnam combat veterans (Table 7.6). We cannot be sure whether this is because Vietnam combat was a more potent stressor overall or because it was simply a more recent one than World War II or Korea. In an A–B–A–B design like this, when differences between the "A"s (wars) appear, they can reflect various phenomena including the age of the respondent, the experiences of the cohort, and (as we have just noted) the recency of the trauma.

CUMULATIVE STRESSORS, THE SELF, AND DISTRESS AMONG WORKING–CLASS MEN

The Stress Process Revisited

In this section, we revisit the stress process and the issue of military service. Our view of this revolves around the concept of identity and related constructs.

Identity. Why should elements of the self like mastery or self–esteem mediate in the stress process? Recent theory has emphasized that the essence of stress lies in the interruption of identity (e.g., Burke, 1991; Burke & Reitzes, 1981, 1991; Riley & Burke, 1995). The experience can become damaging because self–related mediators exist and because they stand between the stressor and the outcome. For example, in Burke's model, stress results when a person perceives a disjunction between the self as one has known it and current feedback about the self. Burke takes a leading role among sociologists who insist on the importance of identity, although his position is relatively extreme in its emphasis on identity interruption; many stressful experiences are not necessarily identity interrupting. Nevertheless, his position need not be literally correct to be important.

Identity Salience. Thoits (1991) also recently utilized identity theory in an attempt to account for the well–known fact that stressors have variable impacts on individuals (Lazarus & Folkman, 1984). Thoits suggests the concept of *identity–relevant stressors* as a solution to this problem. The idea is straightforward. A stressor should have an impact on the person to the extent that it is relevant to that person's identity (or identities). Her operational definition may, however, be unnecessarily restrictive. Thoits argues that "ex–roles" (roles one no longer occupies) do not have a direct effect on distress; she argues that past identities ("ex–roles") have an indirect influence in the present because they alter the ways in which a person occupies current roles. Unlike Thoits, we expect that stressful events that occurred in the past can directly influence current stress processes, although an identity–relevant ex–role was active. The particular past stressor we have in mind is military combat.

The particular contribution offered by an examination of mastery and self–esteem is the chance to expand upon the notion of *carryover stress*. If the impact of a stressor like combat or joblessness depends on the level of mastery and self–esteem, or vice versa, it represents a new wrinkle on the concept of carryover effects (e.g., Thoits, 1995). To find that a prior stressor affects mastery or self–esteem, which in turn affects depression, would represent *carryover through the self*; the self's constructs about itself mediate between old and new stressful experiences. On the other hand—and not necessarily inconsistent with the first—we may see that there are significant interactions of combat with mastery or self–esteem in predicting distress. The latter amounts to *carryover moderated by the self*.

These various processes may explain differences among forms of distress regarding carryover. For example, it is particularly appropriate for simple carryover effects from combat to a later stressor (i.e., effects of the first type above) to involve anxiety. After all, the disorder most characteristically associated with combat—posttraumatic stress disorder (PTSD)—is an anxiety disorder. Intensification of anxiety among the combat veteran can be easily seen as an instance of situational activation spurred by hypervigilance. The person is not continually distressed, but is alert, and when a new stressor is identified, the alarms that go off inside this person's head are louder than they would be without the combat experience. It is less clear that elements of the self should mediate or moderate between other factors and anxiety. Anxiety is a kind of diffuse fear. To be afraid does not require complex involvement of (mediation through or moderation by) the self. It simply requires that men, or women, or dogs, or pigeons, be reminded of a circumstance that once meant fear.

The situation may be different for depression. Depression is a form of distress that is intimately related to mastery and self–esteem to the extent that some clinical discussions make one or both of these self–views not just precursors to but part of the very definition of depression (Beck, 1967; but see Pearlin et al., 1981). In other words, feeling efficacious and believing that one has worth may not only *predict* being undepressed; they may be part of what it *means* to be undepressed. Chapter Eight will return to the elements of depression in greater depth. In the meantime, it is obvious that mastery and self–esteem should be good predictors of depression, and therefore they may mediate the effects of various other factors. And if there is an interactive (moderator–type) carryover effect from combat, it appears plausible to find it in the path from the self to depression by way of mastery and self–esteem. We expected that one or both of the second and third forms of carryover summarized before would emerge for depression.

In the language of quasi–experiments (see Chapter Two), hostility is a kind of "control group" against which the other forms of distress can be compared. We expected and earlier found that combat veterans are more hostile than other men. This is a result even simpler than a carryover: A main effect suggests that the combat veteran is still responding to the original stressor or its sequelae, decades later, regardless of the presence or absence of new stress. It is perhaps more accurate to term this a *carry–on* of early stressful experience. Hostility did not show an interaction with either joblessness or financial hardship (a simple carryover) earlier. What we will explore here is whether the continuous interpersonal consequences that hostility generates may seep into the self, so that mastery or self–esteem either mediates or moderates the stress process for hostility.

Anxiety and hostility are matters of fear and anger. This chapter's continued search for carryover stress may implicate depression to a greater extent than the last chapter because our focus is on carryover stress mediated or moderated by the self. Unlike anxiety and hostility, depression is intimately linked to self–worth, self–control, self–blame, and all the other intimately self–related elements of distress.

Combat and the Self: Prior Carryover Studies. Two studies of Vietnam veterans ask questions similar to ours, but it is difficult to draw firm conclusions from the findings (Ritter, 1984; Vinokur et al., 1987). In each case, the current stressor pertains to job strains or disruptions, and a prior stressor is military combat. Vinokur et al. (1987) also explored main and interactive effects of other early life experiences (e.g., troubled childhood and adolescence). Vinokur et al. (1987) found that prior combat was associated with greater distress during current job disruption, but Ritter (1984) did not. Conversely, Ritter observed an interaction between combat and current job strains, but Vinokur et al. found no interactions between combat and either current or prior stressors. Part of the inconsistency may be due to divergent ways of defining or measuring the variables. Ritter's independent variable was "job strain" rather than "unemployment"; Vinokur et al.'s dependent variable was an omnibus combination of anxiety, depression, and self–esteem, meaning that the relationships among these constructs could not be studied. Such divergences are closer to the rule than the exception in research on combat and indeed in research on stress more generally. In any case, these studies show that combat has either a main effect or an interactive effect on later distress (or both).

Overall, we had expected to find that having occupied the role of soldier, and especially having been in combat, would increase distress directly and would work indirectly or interactively through the self to modify the stress response. The first of these expectations has already been borne out. Now we turn to the second.

Results

We moved sequentially through the steps of the causal model outlined in Chapter One (Figures 1.1 through 1.6) using ordinary least squares (OLS) regressions.

Table 7.7 summarizes the full causal model for men's depression.

Table 7.7 shows no direct effects of joblessness on either mastery or self–esteem once financial hardship is taken into account. Financial hardship, in

Table 7.7
Carryover Stress and the Self:
Prior Combat, Current Joblessness, and Depression Among Male Autoworkers [a]

	Financial Hardship	Mastery	Self–esteem	Depression
Current stressor				
Joblessness	13.93[c]	.01	−.31	.75[c]
	(2.41)	(.05)	(.17)	(.21)
Mediators and moderators				
Social support (Married)	.46	−.02	.06[b]	−.09[b]
Coping (spouse employed)	2.49	−.00	−.00	.05
Financial hardship	——	−.005[c]	−.001[c]	.002[c]
Mastery	——	——	.36[c]	−.16[c]
Self–esteem	——	——--	——	−.46[c]
Jobless x Mastery	——	——	.09	−.20[c]
Prior stress				
Military	−1.92	.04	−00	−.55
Combat	3.92	−.02	.01	1.33[c]
Military x self–esteem	——	——	——	.14
Combat x self–esteem	——	——	——	−.34[c]
Initial Depression	——	——	——	.25[c]
Intercept	93.85	3.71	2.20	3.12
R^2 =	.29	.12	.38	.54

[a] N=863. Interactions of joblessness with all mediators and of the social support and coping variables with joblessness and with all other mediators were tested; as shown above, only the joblessness–mastery interaction attained significance at the p < .01 level. Interactions of military and combat with joblessness and with all mediators were also tested; only the self–esteem interaction shown above was significant at p < .01. All models included age, race, education, prior income, and other negative life events as controls.
[b] p < .05.
[c] p < .01.

Table 7.8
Relationship of Joblessness to Depression
by Levels of Mastery [a]

	Not Employed	Employed
Mastery Quartiles (Low to High):		
1	1.53	1.79
2	1.41	1.56
3	1.37	1.41
4	1.35	1.35

[a] Cells show mean depression scores on 1–5 scale, where 5=highest depression. Means are taken from an analysis of covariance in which all main effects shown in Table 7.2 were controlled.

turn, affects mastery and self–esteem (both directly and indirectly, through mastery). Financial hardship also increases depression directly, so that the greater the financial hardship, the more severe the depression. Overall, the paths of influence from financial hardship to depression are many: a direct trail, an indirect effect through self–esteem, an indirect effect through mastery, and an indirect effect through both mastery and self–esteem in sequence.

The original Pearlin et al. (1981) stress model emphasized the potential importance of social support and of coping strategies in alleviating depression; each of these forces can play a dual role, either as main effects or as moderators of the rest of the stress process. Table 7.7 shows that our measure of economic coping (spousal employment) had no effects and our measure of social support (marriage) had only direct effects on self–esteem and depression (increasing the former and decreasing the latter). Only one interaction involving the current stressor—that between joblessness and mastery in predicting depression—was significant. The average level of depression at different levels of mastery indicated that unemployment accentuated the relationship between mastery and depression. (See Table 7.8.) In practical terms, this means that joblessness and low mastery form a "double whammy" associated with higher depression.

Earlier Stressors: "Ex–Roles"

We expected that men's military and combat experience would be the source of carryover stress involving the self.

Both Tables 7.7 and 7.9 address the question of long–term effects of combat on men's depression. First, Table 7.7 showed that combat had a direct effect on depression. Men who had experienced combat were significantly more depressed than others. In addition, combat interacted with self–esteem in much the same way joblessness interacted with mastery. Table 7.9 reports average depression scores at varying levels of self–esteem and employment status. Combat experience accentuated the effect of self–esteem on depression; low self–esteem among combat veterans was associated with particularly high depression.

Results for anxiety and hostility were far less rich. Combat experience did not interact with self–esteem, but it did interact with mastery in predicting anxiety. To be a combat veteran meant an accentuated effect of mastery on anxiety. We have suggested that a linkage of mastery and anxiety is particularly appropriate because at its core, to be anxious is to fear not being able to cope, to succeed, to master an environment. So anxiety destroys mastery and mastery alleviates anxiety.

Hostility, in contrast, did not interact with either of the aspects of the self. It was related to few other things at all, with one stubborn exception: combat veterans were more hostile. It is not necessary to imagine any complex series of disorders, traumas, and the like to make sense of this. In fact, it helps to make sense of one apparently incongruous result encountered earlier with the full sample: on the whole, women were more hostile than men. This need not mean women were more violent—only that they were more pressed by their environment to the extent they wanted to, but probably did not, hit back. Similarly, combat veterans, more than their fellow men, felt more pressed. In our view, both of the hostile groups fit a profile which says that continuous environmental pressure—a tough life in which one bad thing leads to another—can "keep alive" a grudge. For women, chronic conditions of life build anger; for combat veterans, chronic memories and the sequelae of war (in life circumstances and in others' reactions) maintain anger.

Of course, it is important to keep these patterns in perspective. The differences between combat veterans and others, or between men and women, were matters of degree, not categorical distinctions. In the terms of Chapter Four, these were not crazy people; they were frightened, angry, and sad.

Table 7.9

Relationship of Military/Combat Experience to Depression
by Levels of Self–Esteem [a]

		No Military Experience	Military, No Combat	Combat
Self–Esteem Quartiles (Low to High)	1	1.75	1.60	1.89
	2	1.42	1.42	1.44
	3	1.37	1.35	1.31
	4	1.29	1.26	1.28

[a] Cells show mean depression scores on 1–5 scale, where 5=highest depression. Means are taken from an analysis of covariance in which all main effects were controlled.

CONCLUSION: EXPLORING THE PROCESS

Mastery. Recent research has made much of the effort that humans make to see themselves as efficacious in their world. Indeed, self–efficacy is increasingly being viewed as a key underpinning of self–esteem (Gecas, 1989). Looked at in this light, our findings of a direct, indirect, and interactive role of mastery in the stress process suggest that the relationship of efficacy and stress is a fruitful one for study. As Burke (1991) argued, we saw a mastery–depression connection: high mastery, low depression. Further, mastery was tied to depression indirectly through self–esteem. High mastery was associated with high self–esteem, and high self–esteem was linked to low depression.

There were also interactive ties. The impact of a current stressor (joblessness) depended upon the level of mastery; the combination of low mastery and joblessness was a particular recipe for disaster. We believe that this interaction is a telling one, because *unemployment itself is likely to harm the sense of efficacy.* Then, on top of what mastery does in the simple main effects or indirect paths of the stress model, a person's sense of mastery or lack thereof may condition the self to respond to a mastery–draining experience (such as joblessness) with active coping, on the one hand, or with apathy, inattention, and despair, on the other.

Self–esteem. Just as mastery and fears of its lack form a leading indicator for depression, self–esteem operated as more of a lagging or long–term indicator. Self–esteem was driven by mastery rather than the reverse, and when self–esteem interacted with a stressor, it did so with a distant rather than an immediate stressor. This set of patterns is consistent with self–esteem being more stable and unmodifiable than mastery (Rosenberg, personal communication). Whatever feelings the men in our study of plant closings had about themselves as a result of their wartime experiences, they had these feelings for a long time.

Combat appears to have remarkably persistent effects. Given that these data were gathered in 1989 (before the Gulf War), the effects of combat we have been witnessing refer, for the most part, to events that occurred somewhere between Dday and the fall of Saigon. These are old battles, but they appear to be fresh in the minds of these men when they tell us about their sense of self–esteem or their feelings of depression. At some level, they point to the permanent impact of certain identity–defining roles on the unfolding life course.

Implications

It is appropriate to note here the ways in which this sample is especially appropriate for investigating combat as a carryover stressor. Blue–collar men traditionally have made up a large portion of the armed forces and especially of Vietnam combat troops (Appy, 1993). Thus it is possible to generalize to a substantial portion of the male population which has experienced military service. Indeed, the limitation of our sample—the fact that all of the men were blue–collar autoworkers—is simultaneously its strength. A large homogenous sample makes it possible to tease out the telltale difference between the men who *served* during a war and the men who *fought* it, a difference that tends to occur in both the World War II/Korea and Vietnam cohorts.

Looked at from a life course perspective, all wars represent an intersection between the military as an institution and the youth who move through that institution. Vietnam differed from World War II and Korea in the way it intersected with the lives of men from different social classes. From this standpoint, the Vietnam era may have been unique for its simultaneous offering of the historically expected financial and educational benefits of military service, benefits traditionally enjoyed as routes to upward mobility for poor and working class men, coupled with the potentially crippling impact of combat in an unpopular war. Blue–collar men disproportionately experienced both the best and the worst that the military as an institution had to offer to Vietnam Era Americans. The blue–collar men who went to work for GM and other automakers after Vietnam had a respite from struggle and stress that was all too short. And then the plants closed.

Economic crises are like wars: They represent an intersection between the economy and the personnel moving into and through that economy. Sociologists need to heed not just the main effects, but also the configurations of stressors that make life experiences a challenge for one person and a crisis for another. For those workers who move through a major downsizing carrying burdens (such as combat memories), lacking resources (as is true of the unmarried), and wearing a shirt with a blue–collar, troubles are not just happening, they are multiplying and cascading. Combinations of time, place, stressors, and personal history make each individual's journey through hard times a unique one; it is our task as sociologists to find the universal in the unique.

8

Psychological Resources and Distress

It used to be that working for GM gave you a sense of meaning. You worked for the number one auto company. What more could you want? But now—after all of this, we have nothing left. GM is the one who has run away from us, but everyone blames us. For what? A reasonable standard of living—one that everyone should have who works in a factory all day?

—a closing plant worker

The whole plant closing thing toughened me up more than it hurt me. Only I probably work a lot harder for a lot less now. But what am I going to do?

—a second worker

In hard times, some workers find a reason to believe in themselves and their futures. Others find despair. What is the difference between those who say, "the whole plant closing thing toughened me up," and those who claim that "everybody blames us"? This chapter provides more pieces of the puzzle.

First, a stocktaking. What do we know already? We showed earlier that there are broad differences in mental health between closing and nonclosing plant workers. Closing plant workers experienced greater depression and anxiety. Because depression emerged as the most lingering of the mental health consequences of plant closing, it is the main focus of this chapter. We also demonstrated that a cycle can arise in which unemployment generates depression, which leads to unemployment, which leads to further depression.

Earlier we documented that certain groups of workers were either generally more susceptible to depression or especially susceptible to the stress of unemployment. We interpreted these patterns in terms of the resources workers could bring to bear to cope with stress. Chapter Six highlighted economic and social factors, particularly race and gender, and tried to show how a person's identities convey different amounts or types of resources in the battle against stress. As the economists would put it, there is economic, cultural, social, and symbolic capital involved in being white as opposed to black, male as opposed to female, and so on.   Chapter Six emphasized what we did find, not what we didn't, but of course, it was not always true that a worker who "should" be depressed or anxious actually was. In other words, trends have exceptions. It was sometimes true that unemployment did not take the toll it "should." And trends in unemployment did not always translate into trends in mental health. For example, some people who were unemployed at one point and stayed unemployed became less depressed rather than more so. Why?

It is clear that certain ingredients—certain of the things that make us all unique—are still missing from the picture. Among them are the *psychological resources* upon which people can draw and the *liabilities* they suffer. A person's psychological strengths are a kind of "symbolic capital" (Bordieu, 1986) that can be "spent" in restoring the world to its original upright position. Conversely, psychological liabilities also have a role in the emotional economy of mental health. Being depressed, In itself, is an excellent example of a liability. Depression colors the person's emotions, thoughts, and behaviors (e.g., Beck 1967, 1987; overview in Gilbert 1992). Depression is not solely "feeling blue" or a set of thoughts inside the head. Depression leads us to deal with our world differently, and much of the time it leads people to act in ways that may make the situation worse. Consider unemployment. Depression may lead to indecisiveness, despair, and therefore inaction and no action is bad action when a new job must be found. Or consider the emotional ties that make our lives worth living—for most people, our own personal reasons to believe. The tragedy here is that depression is not just personal, but interpersonal. There is an awful symmetry to the idea of having a conversation. Every time a depressed person has a conversation with a loved one, the loved one is having a conversation with—and coping with—a depressed person. As an old song put it, "smile and the world smiles with you, cry and you cry alone." Depressed people are poor company. Only recently, in fact, have social scientists begun to demonstrate that some of the troubles of depressed people are outgrowths of their own behaviors (Coyne, 1992).   In our terms, depression is a liability. Depression invites the fates to make a self–fulfilling prophecy of the person's depressed moods and thoughts and it seals the prophecy with the person's deeds.

Therefore, in exploring the question of workers' psychological resources, we chose to focus on why some people became less depressed as the panel survey progressed, whether or not it seemed that they "should." One important reason might be the simple fact that depressions do go away on their own. But part of the reason, we suspected, might be other psychological resources. This chapter highlights two of these: workers' *coping strategies* and their ability to avoid *self–blame*.

STRESS AND COPING REVISITED

Earlier chapters have talked about job loss as an example of what social scientists call the "stress process." Part of that process is the coping in which the person engages to try to deal with the situation. In social science, the study of coping has been dominated by the cognitive model of Lazarus & Folkman (1984; but for further discussion, see also Coyne & Lazarus, 1980; Folkman, 1984; Folkman & Lazarus, 1985; Goldberger & Breznitz, 1982; and Hobfoll, 1988, 1989; and Lazarus, 1966). In this model, the person has to answer certain questions about what is happening, and these answers help to shape the coping response. According to Lazarus & Folkman (1984, p. 31), a *primary appraisal* is a person's answer to the question, "Am I in trouble or being benefited, now or in the future, and in what way?" A *secondary appraisal* asks, "What if anything can be done about it?" Coping can be cognitive or behavioral—can involve thoughts or deeds—and refers to "efforts to manage specific external and/or internal demands that are appraised as taxing or exceeding the resources of the person" (Lazarus & Folkman, 1984, p. 141).

People may characteristically try to cope in one way more than another, and different situations may call for different kinds of coping responses. Types of coping can be broadly characterized as *problem–focused* versus *emotion–focused* (Folkman & Lazarus, 1980; Lazarus & Folkman, 1984). As the names suggest, problem–focused coping is directed toward managing the problem itself; emotion–focused coping is directed toward managing one's emotional response to that problem.

Coping: Expectations and Outcomes

In our surveys, the questions that were asked in the latter two waves about the person's employment status and plans make it possible for us to think of employment status as a *decision* about whether to look for work (a problem–focused action) or not to do so and to see how this relates to depression and change in depression. The psychological puzzle has three pieces:

the *objective situation* (am I employed or unemployed?)

the *action implications of that situation* (looking for work or not?)

and the *concrete outcome* (did I get what I wanted or not?).

What becomes crucial from this perspective is not just "objective reality" but also the worker's view of that reality, and what it means for him or her. From a worker's viewpoint, having a job may not always be what's best. Reemployment is sometimes stressful, especially if the job obtained is not a good one or not as good as what went before (Liem & Liem, 1988). On the other hand, to be without a job need not be stressful unless a person is seeking work and not finding it (Kessler et al., 1987a, b).

More generally, in the language of stress research, to exercise—or attempt to exercise—control over a situation need not be always beneficial (Folkman, 1984). When a situation is truly controllable, problem–focused action is called for and pays off for mental health, but when a situation is truly uncontrollable, emotion–focused coping may have better consequences for mental health.

As outlined earlier in the book, seven different categories of labor force participation could be distinguished on the basis of the survey's questions about activities and plans. Here we reintroduce them, adding in our inferences about what we think they meant in terms of workers' appraisals of their situation:

1. Working for GM (situation not threatening, no action called for).

2. Working for new employer, not looking for work (situation not threatening, no action called for).

3. Working for new employer, looking for work (situation threatening, action called for).

4. Unemployed, temporarily not looking for work (situation somewhat threatening, no action called for).

5. Unemployed, looking for work (situation threatening, action called for).

6. Unemployed, discouraged worker not looking for work (situation highly threatening, incapacitated from action).

7. Retired (situation not threatening, no action called for).

The main theoretical question about coping decisions concerns change in depression as a function of coping behavior. To reduce the possibility that workers' announced coping decisions were simply rationalizations of current circumstances, we use Wave 2 coping decisions as predictors of change in depression by Wave 3. In terms of coping choices, the active and problem–focused coping step is to look for work (groups #3 and #5 above). Looking may, of course, be accompanied by more emotion–focused coping such as reevaluating the type of work that is acceptable. Inaction—not looking for work—is a more ambiguous way of coping that can be problem–focused, emotion–focused, or both. Its meaning depends on context. Workers who plan to continue at their original employer (#1 above) or at a new employer (#2) are expressing at least a certain level of satisfaction. They are *voluntarily not looking* for work. Retirement and discouragement represent different reasons for inaction. Retirement (#7 above) involves the worker's saying that the working/not working distinction no longer applies. Retirees may be relatively satisfied. And finally, discouraged workers (#6) are showing clear evidence of the strain of unemployment.

Among unemployed workers, only one group could be said to be "voluntarily–not–looking" for work: Group 4, who declared themselves to be temporarily out of the labor force, but said they were not discouraged and were not retired.

To sum up, we expected that "getting better" would be a matter of the fit between the job situation as the worker defined it at Wave 2 and the job situation as it unfolded by Wave 3. In short, if what you get is what you expected to get and it's a job, that should relieve depression. But if you get what you expected, even if that is *not* having a job, it is something for which you have prepared. You can cope with it.

Starting Points

First we looked at patterns of depressive symptoms for each of the seven employment categories just discussed, as of the second and third surveys in the panel study. Figure 8.1 shows these trends.

First we take a hard look at Wave 2 depression levels for each employment category, checking whether the differences between the groups are consistent with what we have speculated was going on—the appraisals we thought were being made. In Fig. 8.1, the first six employment groups from left to right are arranged in what we thought would be, roughly, least distressed (those still working at GM) to most distressed (discouraged workers). We thought the seventh group, retirees, would be relatively low in distress. The figure confirms these expectations. It appears that—from left to right—groups 1, 2, and 7 felt that they were in more or less equal (and relatively good) situations. And groups 3, 4, and 5 felt that they were in more or less equal (and relatively bad) situations. Finally, group 6 (discouraged workers) had things the worst.

Depression and the Fit between Expectation and Reality

Instead of focusing on the left to right differences among groups in Fig. 8.1, let us now shift to the up and down dimension, the differences between the line that signifies Wave 2 scores and the line that depicts Wave 3 scores. In general, as was to be expected, the line for Wave 3 was lower than that for Wave 2. Depressions do go away. But where was there significant change? First let us document its absence. In four of the seven groups, in fact, there was no significant change across the surveys. Three groups had initially low levels of symptoms which remained low. These were the workers who

were still at GM (#1)

had new jobs that they were not looking to leave (#2) or

were retired (#7).

And one group (#6), which initially had high levels of symptoms, also did not show significant change, the discouraged workers. (Despite the fact that Fig. 8.1 shows what looks like a decline in depression for this group, there were so few of them—only 7 people—that this decline was not statistically significant.)

Meaningful, measurable change happened in three places in Figure 8.1.

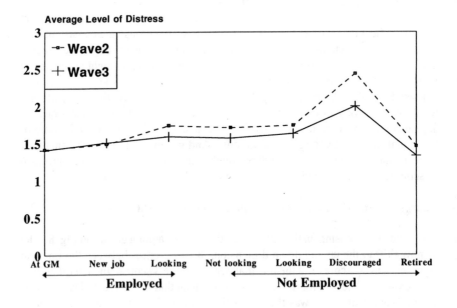

Figure 8.1. Wave 2 and Wave 3 symptoms of depression by worker's Wave 2 self–categorized employment situation.

Depression dropped significantly between Wave 2 and Wave 3 for three of the groups whose Wave 2 level of depression had been relatively high. These were workers who, as of Wave 2

had jobs but were looking for other ones (#3)

were unemployed and not temporarily looking for work (#4) or

were unemployed and actively looking (#5).

Understanding Change in Depression

What makes people less depressed? From the three groups listed previously, whose depression symptoms declined by the end of the study, one might guess that there is a simple explanation. Maybe they got jobs (or better jobs), whether or not they said they wanted them. This explanation relies entirely on an objective resource, jobs. It is possible to test this explanation by incorporating these three groups into a systematic comparison among four employment categories:

new job, satisfied (not looking) as of Wave 2 (#2)

new job, dissatisfied (looking) (#3)

unemployed, temporarily not looking (#4)

unemployed, looking for work (#5).

Logically, these four groups represent all possible combinations of having/not having new jobs and being satisfied/dissatisfied with their situations. Psychologically, all of these groups had been touched by unemployment in some way, and they all described their coping decision as a voluntary choice, whether the choice was action or inaction (Folkman, 1984; Mirowsky & Ross, 1990; Seligman, 1975).

The issue for these four groups is whether depression as of Wave 3 is linked to how these workers saw their situations a year earlier or whether it simply reflects the jobs they had by that point. We can see which explanation is better by dividing the four groups further into those who did and didn't have jobs at Wave 3, and then checking for trends in depression.

Table 8.1 shows the results. Comparisons between the first and second columns establish the trends in depression across waves among those who were *employed* as of Wave 3. Comparisons between the third column and the fourth show the trends in depression for those who were *not employed* at Wave 3.

Depression dropped significantly between Wave 2 and Wave 3 for two of the eight groups that now existed:

unemployed workers who were looking for jobs and found one

unemployed workers who were not looking for jobs and didn't find them.

In addition, a small group of 13 workers who had jobs as of Wave 2 but were looking for other jobs, and then lost (or quit) the jobs by Wave 3, also became less depressed. This trend was not quite statistically significant at our usual standard (p < .05).

It matters what people think is going on, what people think are their goals. Of course, if you are unemployed, seeking work actively, and find it, you feel better. No social scientist would predict otherwise. But it also appears to be true that if you *don't* want work and *don't* find it, you also feel better. In fact, your depression symptoms drop even more sharply if you don't find work than if you do. And to leave a job that was making you unhappy, not surprisingly, makes you happier.

Of course, employment matters. The worker's coping decisions also matter.

What Shapes the Meaning of Jobs?

People do not decide randomly either that they are satisfied with what they have or that they must seek to change it. Yet in the discussions so far, in looking at the way workers coped with their job situations, we have not been taking into account workers' personal characteristics. It is difficult to do so, because some of the employment categories are so small. But we can at least describe each group's characteristics, hoping that it can help to shed light on where different coping decisions come from. After all, it is these same characteristics—race and gender and education and so forth—that earlier chapters emphasized serve as "resources" and as "capital" for overcoming the stress of unemployment. Workers' personal characteristics are the social structural roots of vulnerability and resistance to stress.

It is important to emphasize that to describe the social structural underpinnings of workers' coping decisions is not somehow to replace "subjective" psychological resources with "objective" social ones. The social structural roots of misery and the personal experience of it occur at different levels of analysis. For example, if a statistical analysis shows that social structural factors completely account for the different patterns of coping decisions, a sociologist might say that these structural variables "explain" the coping. But it would be just as accurate to say that the different coping decisions are the ways in which social structurally generated resources and liabilities play themselves out in daily life.

Table 8.2 summarizes seniority and other personal characteristics for the most important of the categories of coping decisions. First, for purposes of comparison, we show a profile of the characteristics of workers who were still at GM as of Wave 3 of the surveys. These are followed by the four key groups (#2–5 earlier) touched by job loss. As before, these represent the four logical combinations among having a new job versus having no job and being satisfied versus being dissatisfied.

All comparisons in this table are tested by t–test or chi–square and are significant at p < .05. Workers who were still at GM were overwhelmingly white males with high seniority. Workers with new jobs, whether or not they were

Table 8.1
Depression at Waves 2 and 3 by Wave 3 Employment Status and Worker's Wave
2 Self–Categorized Employment Situation [a]

Self–Categorization	Wave 3 Employed		Wave 3 Not Employed	
	Depression Wave 2	Depression Wave 3	Depression Wave 2	Depression Wave 3
Wave 2 employed				
New job	1.48	1.50	1.61	1.56
	(89)	(89)	(3)	(3)
New job, looking	1.69	1.57	1.90	1.64
	(45)	(45)	(13)	(13)
Wave 2 unemployed				
Looking	1.68	1.50[c]	1.81	1.77
	(95)	(95)	(89)	(89)
Not looking	1.62	1.53	1.76	1.59[b]
	(42)	(42)	(69)	(69)

[a] $N = 445$; category N's appear in parentheses below each mean. Analyses do not control for demographic factors.
[b] Different from Wave 2 depression (the mean to its immediate left) at $p < .05$ by dependent t–test.
[c] $p < .01$.

satisfied with them, were younger, had less seniority, and more education than workers who remained at GM. Perhaps the most interesting comparisons involve the unemployed workers those who defined themselves as temporarily unemployed versus those who were looking for jobs. Temporarily unemployed workers had more seniority and were older than those who were looking. Both of these groups, in turn, were more often female and were less educated than the workers who had found new jobs that they liked.

For the reader's information, the 35 retired workers (not shown) were, not surprisingly, much older and had more seniority than other groups, and they were the least well–educated. Otherwise they resembled workers still at GM in being overwhelmingly white, male, and married, and having a similar prior incomes. The tiny discouraged worker category ($N = 7$) was diametrically different from retirees in most respects. Compared to the rest of the sample, these workers were disproportionately female, unmarried, had high seniority, were older, and had a low level of education and of initial income.

These numbers tell us something about who took which strategies for dealing with the bad hand these workers were dealt. It also offers some insight into the reasons why they might have done one thing or another. Just as we showed earlier how it can be rational to be depressed in hard times, these profiles of who made which choices make good hard rational sense. In particular, the relatively high seniority of the workers who said they were voluntarily out of the labor force (group 4) helps us to see these workers as rational, utility maximizers. Having more

Table 8.2
Major Self–Categorized Employment Statuses:
Workers' Personal Characteristics [a]

$N =$	Employed Wave 2			Unemployed Wave 2	
	At GM	New Job	Looking	Not Looking	Looking
	591	92	58	111	185
Categorical variables					
Minority (%)	18.8	30.4	19.0	29.7	29.3
Female (%)	9.0	18.5	34.5	41.4	37.5
Married (%)	83.2	67.3	67.2	68.5	56.5
Continuous variables:					
Seniority	18.8	7.3	8.9	14.0	11.1
Education	12.4	12.6	12.4	12.2	12.0
Age	44.2	36.0	35.3	40.4	38.6
Prior income	43.8	36.7	38.5	39.7	37.8

[a] Dichotomous measures (minority, female, and married) are percentages and the column variable is treated as the independent variable. Seniority, education, and age are measured in years and the worker's prior personal income in thousands of dollars. Data were obtained in Wave 1. All row differences are significant at $p < .05$.

seniority, more hope of returning to a job whose pay they could not match elsewhere, they could and did decide, "I'm waiting." It was rational for workers whose contractual benefits gave them some "breathing room" to use that room to take the chance to wait for a recall to GM. They may also have been aware that other employers were reluctant to hire them because of the probability that they would be recalled to GM jobs. In any event, their behavior is consistent with the idea that *not* acting can be as problem–focused as acting.

Those who had less seniority, and less hope of returning to GM were more likely to decide, "I'm looking." Either way, the important ingredient psychologically may be that the worker can come out feeling like a winner. One way you win by finding a job. The other way you win by not having to give in and take a job that signifies you are on a downward spiral through life.

Some issues in this analysis demand discussion. As Hamilton et al. (1993) note, the uneven and occasionally small cell sizes meant that it was necessary to collapse across one of the between–subject's dimensions in analyzing covariance. Restricting the analysis to workers in groups 2–5 of the employment categories, we included as between–subject's variables the worker's Wave 2 coping decision (looking/not looking) and Wave 3 employment status (i.e., the analysis collapsed across Wave 2 employment status). Wave 2/3 depression was the dependent variable in the repeated measures design. The seven covariates included the workers' personal characteristics and seniority. As in the analyses reported in the text, meaningful change in depression was concentrated among workers who were looking for jobs at Wave 2 and employed at Wave 3 (adjusted $M = 1.69$ and 1.53, respectively) and, conversely, those who were not looking for jobs at Wave 2 and were not employed at Wave 3 (adjusted $M = 1.74$ and 1.58).

Summing Up: Expectations and Outcomes

It must be remembered that for many workers, their own mental health is not the driving force keeping them in jobs or forcing them to seek them. Financial exigencies—bills to pay and mouths to feed—may lead workers to stay in jobs, however depressing they are. Our results simply show how combinations of what workers wanted and what workers got affected trends in depression.

These results should not be viewed as evidence that workers get better by somehow fooling themselves, providing an illusion of control rather than the real thing (for relevant discussions, see Abramson et al., 1978; Bandura, 1977; 1986; Langer, 1983; Mirowsky & Ross, 1990; and Seligman, 1975). Obviously, workers who announce (to the interviewer and to the self) that "I am not looking for a job just now" are providing themselves with a measure of perceived control over the situation, but they also may be generating later actual control. They *cannot* lose (i.e., by failing to get jobs, since they do not want them). They *can* win, first in the simple sense of "buying time" to emerge from depression, and second in the more instrumental ways that were available in this case (e.g., by obtaining retraining, going back to school, and the like). This seems to us more instrumental than illusory.

To lose control of life's direction is depressing. To eke out some sense of control over a life gone haywire eases the burden. You feel less crazy. In these circumstances, rational choices are choices that offer a sense of control over a world gone wrong.

COLLECTIVE WOES AND INDIVIDUAL SELF–BLAME

When plants close, the unemployment that follows is an example of a "fateful loss," the kind of blow over which people have no control, no ability to ward off, and often little psychological protection against (Dohrenwend et al., 1978; Shrout, Link, Dohrenwend, Skodol, Stueve, & Mirotznik, 1989). There is an irony hidden here. The fact that in a plant closing, the unemployment flows from the employer's decision to shut down, and not from the worker's personality or actions, offers one psychological benefit, however modest. Workers whose plants close are not likely to blame themselves for their predicament.

The crux of the matter is not solely what happened to these workers in some objective sense but also *what the workers thought what was happening to them and how they felt about it.* Only by entering their subjective worlds can we grasp what gives some workers reasons to believe in themselves and their tomorrows. Ironically, one source of help proves to be GM, for it offered workers a villain for the drama that was unfolding in their lives. Following, we discuss what workers saw as GM's responsibility and how they saw the larger social context of plant closings.

Job Loss without Self–Blame

As Chapter Two first noted, certain questions were asked only in closing plants in the Wave 1 interview. For example, closing plant workers were asked whether they agreed or disagreed (and, then, whether they "strongly agreed" or "strongly disagreed") with five statements about blame for job loss.

Table 8.3 shows the wording of these questions and the pattern of answers. In each case, workers *denied* that they were to blame. (In four cases, this denial involved disagreeing with the statement. In one case, an "agree" rather than a "disagree" response indicated low self–blame.) Thus, when they were asked directly about whether they felt blameworthy, closing plant workers firmly said "no."

There was a second, less intrusive way of getting at what workers thought. Before answering the questions in Table 8.3, the closing plant workers were asked to give a free response to a question about "who or what you feel is primarily responsible for your job situation." The question about responsibility was both more subtle and potentially more revealing than the questions shown in Table 8.3 because its open–ended format allowed the workers to put into their own words how they felt about their predicament. Up to three answers per worker were coded according to a detailed coding scheme. Overall, we coded 1,321 responses from 812 workers. For present purposes, the most important issue is whether any answers seemed to be self–blaming (such as, "I should have seen this coming and found another job").

Workers' answers varied more in their texture than in their ultimate target. Some answers were abrupt, almost dismissals of the question:

"GM"

"Management"

Other answers conveyed a sense of having personalized the battle:

"Roger Smith and his boys"

"Imports and Roger Smith with his sorry ass, poor management. You can't sell cars that look alike — Riviera, Toronado, Seville, Eldorado — and expect the public to eat it up."

Other answers offered a more complex picture, but still honed in on GM:

Basically the plant is obsolete. That's the reason that they are giving for it. But we are the number one body shop in GM and to have the number one body shop why would you move all of these people to start the same operation somewhere else? Management seems to have a lack of foresight. Management had said that if we get the quality up they

Table 8.3
Responses to General Blame Items by Closing Plant Workers at Wave 1 [a]

Item	Strongly Agree (%)	Somewhat Agree (%)	Somewhat Disagree (%)	Strongly Disagree (%)
Losing this job is due to circum–stances or factors beyond my control	90.8	5.0	1.0	3.3
Others who are important to me blame me for losing this job	1.1	1.6	8.4	88.9
Losing this job is due to some–thing I did or didn't do that I might be able to change in the future	2.3	2.7	8.3	86.6
I blame myself for losing this job	1.3	.7	6.5	91.5
Losing this job is due to the kind of person I am	1.1	.4	6.6	92.0

[a] N ranges from 816 to 822 workers and excludes don't know responses.

would keep it open. They even made a number of improvements. They at one time had a lead contamination problem in the body area. They moved this job to another plant. But they are still going to have the same problem there. So it doesn't make sense to close our plant and move our jobs. However, the plant is obsolete.

And what about self–blame? There was almost none to be found. Originally, we intended to analyze differences between workers who blamed themselves and workers who blamed some other sources for their job situation. Table 8.4, which summarizes the first answers workers gave to the question, shows that this analysis was impossible. Too few workers blamed themselves for any kind of comparison of "self–blamers" with others to be feasible. Only two of these first responses, the first things that came to workers' minds, were self–blaming answers. In fact, only 2 out of the total of 1,321 coded responses were self–blaming—and one of these carried a mixed tone of regret and a sense that a personal contract had been violated:

"I had a goal and I thought that if I went to work every day and did as I was told, everything would be OK."

Clearly, workers perceived responsibility as lying primarily at the door of GM and on the shoulders of its executives. Relatively few answers were negative toward the workers or the union. Few answers were uncodable (confused or off the point). As the table shows, a somewhat larger number focused on the more abstract targets of the economy or foreign competition, but these were dwarfed by the number that zeroed in on GM. Most of the workers made rather global statements in which they attributed the plant closings to a source *external* to themselves, an impersonal and stable cause, rather than to some fleeting source such as bad luck. In plain English, it was GM's fault.

SELF–BLAME AND DISTRESS (ESPECIALLY DEPRESSION)

To the extent that self–blaming itself contributes to poor mental health (Janoff–Bulman, 1979; Peterson, Schwartz, & Seligman, 1981) or is an element of depression (Beck 1967, 1987), workers may be less depressed when a plant closes than when they lose jobs in some other way.

Traditional approaches to defining depression assign a large role to self–blame. Freud, for example, had this to say about what he called "melancholia":

The most striking feature of this illness, of whose causation and mechanism we know much too little, is the way in which the super–ego — "conscience," you may call it, quietly — treats the ego. While a melancholic can, like other people, show a greater or lesser degree of severity to himself in his healthy periods, during a melancholic attack his super–ego becomes over–severe, abuses the poor ego, humiliates it and ill–treats it, threatens it with the direst punishments, reproaches it for actions in the remotest past which had been taken lightly at the time — as though it had spent the whole interval in collecting accusations and had only been waiting for its present access of strength in order to bring them up and make a condemnatory judgment on their basis. (1960)

In the traditional view, self–blame often represents anger turned inward. Anger that

Table 8.4

Closing Plant Workers' Open–Ended Responsibility Answers, Wave 1 [a]

Category	Percent Choosing (N in parentheses)
GM, general or vague	16.9 (137)
Roger Smith specifically mentioned	11.9 (97)
GM, intentionality attributed	16.6 (135)
GM, mismanagement	15.6 (127)
GM, plant level management	3.8 (31)
GM, plants obsolete	4.2 (34)
Workers, union	5.7 (46)
Shared responsibility	6.8 (55)
Economic forces, competition	16.0 (130)
Self to blame	.2 (2)
Self *not* to blame	.4 (3)
Uncodable	1.8 (15)

[a] N = 812 workers; an additional 394 gave a second response, and 115 gave a third response. Their distributions were similar to that shown here, except that no additional self–blaming or self–defending answers were offered.

for some reason cannot or will not be directed at its rightful target is turned upon the self.

Recent theorists agree that depressed people blame themselves but rarely talk of a superego that does the blaming. For example, Beck's highly influential theory of depression focuses on three kinds of thoughts that depressed people have about themselves: a negative view of the self, a negative view of the world as one currently sees it, and a negative image of the future. The negative view of self is permeated with self–blaming. Self–blame is such a universal part of the picture of depression that the main argument among the professionals concerns whether self–blame is a *cause* of depression or a key *element* in it, part of the very definition of what it means to be depressed (Abramson et al., 1978; Abramson, Metalsky, & Alloy, 1989; Beck, 1967, 1976, 1987; Beck, Rush, Shaw, & Emery, 1979; and Haaga, Dyck, & Ernst, 1991).

If self–blame causes depression, then research should show that blaming the self when things go wrong is bad for mental health. However, the actual picture is more complicated. A recent review by Tennen & Affleck (1990) notes that some studies have found that people who blame themselves for various personal tragedies, such as accidents in which they become paraplegic or rapes in which they are victims, adjust *better* than those who do not self–blame. These studies were attention–getting precisely because they flew in the face of the accepted wisdom about blame and mental health. Yet this review suggests that people have drawn the wrong conclusions: What is important isn't so much self–blame or the absence of self–blame, but whether the person lays blame for misfortunes on other people. Passing the buck—blaming others for one's misfortunes—is associated with poorer adjustment.

But even this new, careful conclusion may need further fine–tuning. Psychologists who study blaming almost always focus on individual traumas for which people blame other individuals. We are faced instead with a collective trauma for which people quite rationally blamed General Motors. We think that the confusing research findings by the psychologists are probably irrelevant to a plant closing. What happens when plants close can be thought of as *a collective depression caused by an impersonal institution*. When we set out to study the plant closings, our gut feeling was that for workers to blame the self in this circumstance was not just harmful to mental health. It was simply nonsense.

Then what is the role of self–blaming in a plant closing? In exploring this issue, we will first set aside for the moment the debate about whether self–blame is a part of depression or one of its causes. Everyone agrees that hand in hand with the other symptoms they have, depressed people tend to blame themselves unduly. We think it is an open question whether the blaming builds the depression or grows out of it. The true answer may be "both of the above."

The remainder of this chapter traces the evidence about self–blame over the three surveys of the panel study, revealing a kind of "natural history" of self blame for a fateful loss. But to understand what we find, it is necessary first to lay a bit more groundwork. Another, potentially competing explanation for depression must be taken into account. This explanation is already familiar. It is the idea that what generates or maintains depression is loss of control. What we plan to do is to patch together the "control" explanation and the "self–blame" explanation to make a simple point: What makes you depressed may not be what keeps you that way.

An Uncontrollable Fate

One alternative theme runs through recent research about depression: the notion that what is important is not self–blame or lack of self–blame but the person's sense of having no control over events. A recent survey by Mirowsky & Ross (1990) showed that the least depressed people were what they called instrumentalists, people who both took credit for successes and accepted blame for failures in their lives. Instrumentalists were less depressed than any of three other groups: (1) fatalists, who took credit for neither success nor failure, (2) self–blamers, who took credit for failure but not success, or (3) self–defenders, who took credit for success but not failure. These authors feel that what causes depression is not self–blaming but the lack of a personal sense of control over one's life.

This view traces back to earlier research by Seligman (1975) in what came to be known as the "learned helplessness" approach to depression. Learned helplessness is something that can be watched in — and taught to — all kinds of animals. Dogs, rats, and people alike have difficulty when negative things happen (stresses, traumas, tragedies). They have great difficulty with uncontrollable events. And they have special troubles with *uncontrollable, negative* events. The "learned helplessness" hypothesis is simple: Lack of control over outcomes generates depression. People fall into depression because they cannot control life's rewards and punishments, not because they think badly of themselves, their situations, and their futures.

More recent versions of the "learned helplessness" argument come close to combining the idea that control is what matters and the idea that self–blame is what matters. Abramson et al, (1978) argued that the person's interpretation of the situation is important. In this view it is a combination of uncontrollability and the person's judgment about where the lack of control came from that creates depression, not life's lack of controllability (or not just that). Depression follows when you combine (1) an uncontrollable event (2) which is negative and (3) whose causes the person sees as "internal, global, and stable." (Internal = I did it. Global = It's something general about me. Stable = I'm always this way.) How can something be uncontrollable, but internally caused? To put it in academic terms, "I failed the test because I'm stupid" implies both an internal cause and an inability to change the outcome. Out in the real world, so does "I didn't leave GM earlier because I'm a jerk." An internal, global, stable attribution for a negative event *is* basically self–blame (Abramson et al., 1989; Sweeney, Anderson, & Bailey, 1986). Putting these together, what recipe for depression do we have? Mix the following:

something negative happens in your life;

it (or repairing it) is beyond your control;

something about you caused it or prevents its cure.

It may not be necessary to have all of these ingredients all of the time. Theories differ. Research hasn't given us final answers. But if all of them are present, they are a potent mix to swallow.

What Does It Mean To Have Depression Without Self–Blame?

When things go wrong, people are motivated to make sense of them, to figure out why they happened. At least some people are likely to think such thoughts as "that was my fault." It is important to appreciate the ways in which a plant closing is not like other bad outcomes of life. As we have emphasized all along, it would be irrational for a worker to blame the self when a plant closes. Therefore, plant closings represent a kind of real–world "laboratory" in which we might find *depression without self–blame*. From Tables 8.3 and 8.4, it is clear that, at first, workers felt almost no self–blame. But later chapters have amply proved that workers affected by the plant closings—who experienced more unemployment—were more depressed than workers whose plants didn't close.

So why is it interesting that these workers experienced depression without self–blame? It may offer a kind of bridge between theories about *what makes people depressed* and theories about *what enables them to get better*. Perhaps there are changes in the nature of depression over time, and maybe self–blame is an ingredient in lingering depressions or more severe depressions. For example, it is easy to imagine that self–blame can be created by failures to cope with the situation, such as by not finding a job.

Collective Troubles and Individual Self–Blame: Findings

At Wave 1, when answering standard questions about blaming the self and when giving an open–ended answer about responsibility, closing plant workers firmly rejected self–blame. But these questions were not asked at later waves of the survey, ironically because there was so much agreement on them that they were not very interesting. Because of their content, they were also not asked of nonclosing plant workers even in the first wave of the survey. But there was one question about self–blame that everyone was asked about in all three surveys. It was one of the 12 depression symptoms, "blaming yourself for things." Using that question, we can compare the closing and nonclosing plant workers and can look for trends over time in self–blame, compared to the other symptoms of depression.

First and foremost, if there is nothing different about self–blame — if it behaves exactly like the other symptoms of depression — then there is no justification for treating it as special, for setting it aside from the other 11 symptoms. So we need to find out if it has any kind of special status.

Table 8.5 shows the average scores for each symptom at Wave 1. The table divides the workers into closing versus nonclosing plants and then further divides the closing plant workers into those who had or had not already lost jobs. We could have simply compared closing versus nonclosing groups or employed versus unemployed workers, but this way it is easy to see the one–two–three progression in frequency of symptoms. Nonclosing plant workers are always in the best position, followed by closing plant workers with jobs, followed by closing plant workers without jobs.

One symptom differs from the other 11. For that symptom, "blaming yourself for things," there is no clear distinction whatsoever among the groups. Everywhere else, the differences among the groups were sizeable, usually so much so that the result could have occurred only 1 in 10,000 times by chance.

There is a sense in which the table simply reconfirms that what we have here is depression without self–blame, at least at Wave 1. But the table also adds some texture to that conclusion. It shows that an event that everyone agrees is an uncontrollable negative event, plant closing, generates other symptoms of depression without activating self–blame.

It is important to make the distinction between ever blaming yourself and

Table 8.5
Elements of Depression Among Autoworkers: Wave 1 Data [a]

Symptom	Closing Plants Unemployed	Employed	Difference Nonclosing	Significant?
Loss of sexual interest or pleasure	1.57	1.49	1.38	Yes
Trouble getting to sleep or staying asleep	2.22	1.92	1.65	Yes
Thoughts of ending your life	1.15	1.13	1.05	Yes
Poor appetite	1.55	1.33	1.23	Yes
Crying easily	1.42	1.33	1.25	Yes
Feeling of being trapped or caught	1.91	1.78	1.52	Yes
Blaming yourself for things	1.60	1.51	1.58	No
Feeling lonely	1.80	1.66	1.47	Yes
Feeling blue	1.98	1.77	1.61	Yes
Worrying or stewing about things	2.26	2.05	1.93	Yes
Feeling no interest in things	1.74	1.62	1.50	Yes
Feeling hopeless about the future	1.98	1.81	1.56	Yes

[a] N = 202 closing plant unemployed, 625 closing plant employed, and 762 nonclosing plant workers. Significance refers to F–test for one–way analysis of variance. For all items, $p < .001$, and for most items, $p < .0001$.

blaming yourself in a way that is linked to the plants closing. It isn't that closing plant workers were unwilling to blame themselves for anything. There is self–blame floating around in Table 8.5, as the absolute size of the numbers testifies. (For example, fortunately, the frequency of suicidal thought was lower than the frequency of self–blaming thoughts.) But those workers who were going through the wrenching, uncontrollable negative event of having their plant close down were not blaming themselves any more than workers who were not.

Trends over Time

If plant closings are really special, self–blaming might also differ from the other 11 symptoms of depression in the way it develops over time. We will review these trends in two ways. First we compare closing and nonclosing plant workers across all three waves of the survey. Then we will turn to look in greater detail at how workers' employment status affected their self–blame, as opposed to the other 11 depression symptoms (averaged together).

Figure 8.2 shows the trends separately for closing versus nonclosing plant workers, in each case taking into account workers' personal characteristics. The figure is derived from adjusted means from a repeated measures analysis of covariance (ANCOVA) in which depression and self–blame constituted one repeated measure, time (three waves) was the second, and the seven covariates were the demographics plus initial seniority at GM. The between–subjects grouping was closing versus nonclosing plant. We observed a series of highly significant effects of measure (depression/self–blame), measure by group, wave by group, wave by measure, and wave by measure by group, as summarized in the text. First, the panel that shows the results for nonclosing plants provides us with a standard. It is our window into what happens in blue–collar workers' lives when the plant stays open. In these plants, self–blame was more common than other symptoms of depression. There was no significant trend over time in either self–blame or the other symptoms. This lack of pattern in depression is what you would expect if these people are not really being touched by this particular form of distress. The fact that self–blaming is fairly common, relative to other symptoms, means little. It may simply mean that it is easier to admit to blaming oneself than it is to admit to being suicidal or even crying. It may even reflect the fact that people who blame themselves are Mirowsky & Ross's (1990) "instrumentalists," seeing themselves as in control of something in their lives. A little self–blame may be a good thing.

In the other panel, closing plant workers show a different pattern of response and recovery. It is clear that for them, something depressing was happening. It is also clear that "something" *was not the same* for self–blame and the other symptoms. Self–blaming started out quite low, below the levels in the nonclosing plants—the opposite of the pattern for all other symptoms. By Wave 2, self–blame rose significantly for closing plant workers, so that it looked like just another "depression symptom." By Wave 3, in keeping with the fact that depressions lift over time and the fact that people who get jobs become less depressed, both self–blame and the other symptoms recede.

Jobs, Expectations, and Accomplishments

What might explain the rise and fall of self–blaming? Based on what we had already seen about coping in this chapter, it is not surprising that we decided to take a look at the role of workers' coping decisions. Recall that for depression as a whole — without distinguishing self–blame from the other symptoms — we have seen already that workers who could consider themselves to have gotten what they wanted were significantly less depressed by Wave 3 than they had been before. Now it is time to see how self–blaming fits into this pattern.

Figure 8.2 already offers some hints about what might have made closing plant workers blame themselves more in Wave 2 than in Wave 1. As early as Chapter Three we saw that unemployment peak at Wave 2, so perhaps something as straightforward as failure to get or keep a job has something to do with the new self–blame. By Wave 2, in fact, workers who did not have jobs *were* more self–blaming than workers who did have them (in contrast to Wave 1, as Table 8.5 showed). But is that the whole story?

It is time to return to workers' self–defined job statuses as we do in Table 8.6. These were of necessity the job statuses as the workers defined them at Wave 2, of course, because the items about job search were not included in the Wave 1 interview. Based on the earlier results, we concentrate on four categories of *changed* job situations: being in a new job and satisfied, being in a new job and looking for another one, being unemployed but temporarily not looking for work, and being unemployed and looking (i.e., groups 2–5). (For completeness, these analyses were carried out on all workers who found themselves in one of these four situations, whether or not they were initially in closing plants. Being in a closing plant *per se* had no impact after Wave 2, independent of its effect on unemployment. Analyses in which we separated out closing plant workers from the relatively few nonclosing plant workers in these categories did not show that the nonclosing plant workers were distinctive).

What happened by Wave 3? Self–blame dropped only a bit, and only among the 13 workers who (a) had new jobs at Wave 2, but (b) were unsatisfied, and then lost or left those jobs by Wave 3. Other symptoms of depression also dropped for this group. The other results mirrored what we found before. Two groups that had been, by their definitions, successes by Wave 3 showed significant decreases in the

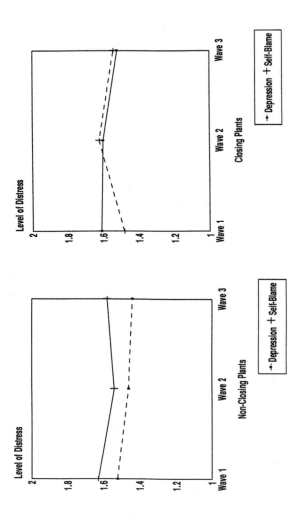

Figure 8.2. Adjusted means for 11–item depression and self–blame: closing and nonclosing plant worker's responses at three waves.

11 depression symptoms: Workers who looked for jobs at Wave 2 and found them, and those who were "unemployed but not looking" and did not get jobs.

Table 8.6
Trends in 11–Item Depression and Self Blame from Wave 1 to Wave 2, by Job
B
Situation at Wave 2 [a]

Job Status	Depression		Self–blame	
	Wave 1	Wave 2	Wave 1	Wave 2
New job (117)	1.52	1.46	1.47	1.57
New job, but looking (70)	1.60	1.71	1.60	1.84[b]
Unemployed, looking (210)	1.68	1.71	1.56	1.70
Unemployed, not looking (130)	1.76	1.70	1.65	1.70

[a] N for each category appears in parentheses beside its label.
[b] Significantly different from the mean to its left at $p < .05$.

Again we see having a job or not having one is not necessarily the driving force behind mental health The issue is whether you have what you want. The results also tell us something about the way a depression that is not initially "attached" to the self by self–blame can change its character over time. In Wave 1, the workers seemed to be experiencing "depression without self–blame." But by Wave 2 self–blame began to attach itself to workers who had failed to get what they wanted — had been unable to find work or to find work that they considered adequate.

Summing Up: Self–Blame

In a plant closing, workers start out able to avoid blaming themselves. Self–blame attaches itself via a worker's perception of having tried to get something and failed. It sticks to its victim. Other symptoms of depression are initially present to a greater degree than self–blame, but these tend to fade away in the face of successes.

These trends enable us to see that there may be a kind of natural history to the way humans respond to an uncontrollable negative event like a plant closing. There may be an initial phase without self–blaming and a later self–blaming phase. The self–blaming grows when the person has not succeeded in coping with the event, *however that person defines coping*, and when the person has failed to meet personal goals, *whatever those goals are*. From this standpoint, each of the alternative theories that emphasize self–blame or lost control in the face of life's traumas speaks a piece of the truth. Depression is "all of the above," and self–blame and perceived lack of control probably work together to maintain it. Self–blame is a bulwark of depression. To exert or assert control and get what you wanted eases self–blame; to exert or assert control and not get what you wanted deepens it. Depression means self–blame for the past, lost control in the present, and lost hope for the future.

CONCLUSIONS

The objective reality of unemployment builds a subjective world for the worker who experiences it. To a significant extent, this is a bleaker world, more colored by depression than the world of the employed worker. Psychological resources for combating depression include how workers decide to cope with the job situation and how they lay blame for their predicament. With regard to coping decisions, this chapter has shown that to make sense of trends in depression over time, it is essential to take the worker's point of view. After all, depression improved noticeably for

workers who wanted jobs and got them,

workers who didn't want jobs and *didn't* get them, and

workers who didn't like their jobs and lost them.

How else would we manage to explain this collection of improvements?

Having a job is not everything. What is important is whether you control—or think you control—what is happening to you. One means of control is to define the situation in a way that works for you. Depression receded when there was a fit between what the worker thought was happening and what did happen, whatever that was.

Of course, there are limits to the magic that can be wrought by redefining goals. Real people are not free to define situations as they see fit, so as to give themselves the most control over their fates. For many workers, their own mental health is not the driving force keeping them in a job or keeping them in the search for one. Bills to pay and mouths to feed may lead workers to stay in jobs, however depressing they are. Our surveys simply show that reality has a little bit of "give" in it, even for an autoworker whose plant just shut down.

Pervasive self–blame is another of the shameful secrets of a depressed mind. We have seen here that the depression associated with plant closing is special in certain ways. Workers start out not blaming themselves in the slightest, but their self–blame grows over time. It grows when they have *failed* to exert control over their fates, by being unable to find jobs or by finding inadequate ones.

This latter result means that plant closings bring with them their own mental health Catch–22. The best way for the worker to pick up the pieces of a shattered work life is to find a new job. But trying — making efforts to get or keep a new job — can bring on self–blame when the efforts fall short. And ultimately the ebb and flow of the economy and the labor force, not the worker, control whether those efforts will or won't fall short.

The end result is what might be called a "plant closing depression." Now we can revisit the words of the worker quoted at the beginning of Chapter Four, recasting them in the language of the theories discussed here:

"Sometimes all I could do was think about what they had done to me. I felt worthless, but mostly I felt it was GM's fault. But there was no GM to

bitch out or get even with."
[The worker showed symptoms of depression — sense of worthlessness, ruminating on the negative event — but was not initially blaming the self.]
"When I couldn't get by any more and I couldn't find a job and I couldn't stand to see anybody I used to work with, I guess I just turned it all on myself."
[The anger turned inward. The worker started self–blaming and isolating the self in response to not being able to gain control of the situation.]
"Yeah, I was crazy."

Sometimes it's normal to be crazy. To demonstrate this fact is not solely an issue for social science. It is a matter of the way individuals, families, and communities are going to cope with a major social dislocation. People whose depressions are severe need help and try to get help. For blue–collar workers, however, it is not always clear that they get the help they need. What they need are jobs. If they get them or if they otherwise avoid self–blaming, the results should fall into line with the typical findings of plant closing research, in which depressions are not very severe and people get better when they get new jobs.

If what workers get is "help" or "support" from others, instead of jobs, our data—like others—indicate that it is much less clear how things will turn out. In particular, Chapter Nine illustrates that the fruits of "seeking professional help" can be more than the worker bargained for.

9

Individual versus Collective Resources

I just couldn't find a job. They didn't want to hire me because I used to make $15.00 per hour. They just would not hire me at $5.00. Things just got rougher and rougher. My relatives helped me out. I almost lost the house. I felt like I was taking handouts. I just keep to myself. I don't want to be around nobody anymore. I don't want to talk to anyone. Things don't look good.

—a divorced woman, living alone

I had nineteen years in when they closed the plant—that's more time in the bathroom than a lot of guys got in seniority. My grandfather was a Sit–Downer back in the thirties. My family's got better than a hundred and thirty years at General Motors. I stayed out two years and then took a transfer out of state. I'd rather be up in Michigan with my family, but what can we do? We have always been from up there and family–wise, this is a big problem. My wife has been behind me a hundred percent, though. I know three different guys I worked with and their wives left them when they took transfers out of state. But, we're doing okay. I just want to get back to Michigan.

—a married man

When a plant closes, people become anxious and depressed. We earlier showed that even workers whose plants *don't* close become anxious. But depression rises where plants do close, and only there. It rises because people lose jobs. It rises particularly among certain groups who lack resources to combat it, whose futures look bleak. And it rises both because of the economic meaning of job loss and, we think, because of the loss of role and loss of standing that unemployment eventually comes to mean.

Chapter Six stressed the tangible resources such as finances that some workers can bring to bear on the problem of survival. When a financial crisis hits, having money helps. Having ways to make more of it also helps. Chapter Six also stressed the mental burden that results from belonging to certain groups that are likely to suffer in the job market. Less educated workers, especially less educated blacks, were more strongly and persistently affected than any other workers by the unemployment they experienced. Chapter Eight explored psychological resources—ways of thinking about the plant closing or the unemployment experience that can help to make each less painful. We saw that how the worker defined his or her job status was as important as what that status was, objectively. Not wanting a job and not getting one were the "moral" equivalent of wanting a job and finding it, at least from the point of view of relieving workers' depression. Either way, it seems, workers were able to reexperience or reexert personal control over a fate that seemingly had gone out of control.

In the light of the findings in Chapter Eight about self–blame versus the other elements of depression, the analyses here use the 11–item version of the scale of depression symptoms of Chapter Eight, which excludes self–blame. Trends for self–blame are considered separately.

This chapter looks further at what makes depressions lift and at what holds self–blame at bay, in other words, at what gives people some reason to believe when a way of life is threatened. If we try to imagine a GM worker at one of the closing plants in 1987 and then follow this worker over the two years during which we kept up with most of them, the factors mentioned thus far only scratch the surface of the things that can give people reason to believe—or that can shake that faith. Neither the objective personal characteristics nor the psychological resources that have been considered so far do much to move away from a picture of the worker as an isolated individual, a body inside a blue–collar. Granted, some of these factors help to give this body a real life in a real social context. For example, we have touched on the impact of marriage and of having someone to confide in. Each of these is a plus, especially in combating depression. We also noted that other negative life events—aside from plant closing and job loss, that is—can also generate depression, anxiety, or both. We will return to the issues of social support and negative life events here.

These and the other themes of the current chapter share one characteristic: They all involve resources *outside the self* on which a worker might draw. These workers had families, friends, fellow religious worshipers, and companions in organizations of all sorts. They had the UAW. And, if they sought it, their health care benefits brought them professional help from generalists or specialists in mental health problems. All of these are potential reasons to believe in the self and in the future.

Of course, these workers were individuals, but individuals are bred and nurtured and healed in networks of others to whom they are tied. Furthermore, the problem these workers faced was at its root a collective problem, not an individual one. Perhaps collective problems are best solved through collective means.

Therefore, this chapter looks to the role of others at several levels in a search for evidence of factors that help mental health, particularly depression. The informal ties of family and friendship, the more formal ties of organizations, and the specific step of seeking professional help might each help build or restore some reason to believe.

We begin by looking at a traditionally individualistic solution to mental health problems, asking and getting help from a professional. This is compared and contrasted with seeking help informally. Then we turn from *seeking* help to *having* help, friends, contacts, and activities. We explore and compare various avenues of social support from the most intimate and informal support (having a confidant) to the most organizational and collective (religious worship and union membership). What the chapter will show is that people do weave reasons to believe from the social fabric of the world around them, and they benefit especially from their intimate and their collective ties.

GETTING HELP: DOES IT HELP?

When you need help for a mental health problem, does it actually help to ask for it? The answer is not as obvious as it seems. There are two issues to be considered here. First, what do we know about the general effect of seeking help—from anyone, for anything? Second, what about the issue of *from whom* the help comes?

The social science literature on helping behavior, particularly in social psychology, has shown that although people often view receiving assistance as beneficial, it is not unlikely that those who seek help also experience many negative consequences from the help–seeking encounter (Fisher, Nadler, & Whitcher–Alagna, 1982). These consequences include feelings of failure, inferiority, and dependency (Fisher & Nadler, 1974). This help–seeking literature suggests that part of the dynamics of seeking help is labeling of oneself as needing the help of others to solve one's problems. Although this literature has not directly dealt with seeking help for troubled mental health, it alerts us to the possibility that seeking help may have the negative outcome of decreasing the sense of personal control.

Informal Help

Given this backdrop, first we looked at a set of questions that workers were asked about whether they had consulted a variety of informal sources of help for

"personal, emotional, behavioral, or mental difficulties, worries, or 'nerves'. . . during the past year. The sources included:
    spouse or partner
    children
    other family members
    co–workers or supervisor
    bartender
    barber or hairdresser
    a stranger.
Recall that we and others have found that being married is associated with less depression, and so is having someone to confide in (which is almost always the spouse, among those who are married). Whatever the labeling and humiliation that seeking help can entail, it should be minimal where one's spouse is concerned. We would expect that help from a spouse shouldn't hurt, and it might help. On the other hand, all informal sources of support are not necessarily equal. People who are telling strangers that they have troubled mental health probably are worse off anyway, and they are not likely to get much assistance from such sources.

      Figure 9.1 shows the Wave 3 depression scores for workers who did or did not seek help during the preceding year from these two extremes—spouse and stranger—among the informal sources of help. (Answers were not mutually exclusive, so those who sought help from strangers may also have sought help from

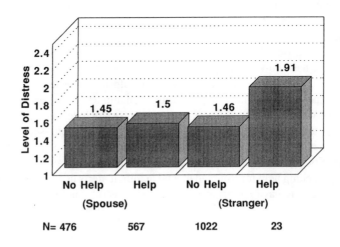

Figure 9.1. Wave 3 depression as related to seeking help informally during the previous year.

spouses and vice versa.)

First, it is important to get a sense of how rare or common it was to turn to each of these sources of help. The figure includes at the bottom the numbers of people in each group to illustrate the fact that many of the choices are quite rare. Thus at the bottom right, we see that in the Wave 3 interview, only 23 workers reported that they had sought help from strangers during the preceding year. Help from spouses, on the other hand, was quite commonly reported. (The other sources of help that we asked about were intermediate between these two, both in their frequency of occurrence and in their apparent effect on depression.)

Given these differences, how was the seeking of help from each source related to subsequent depression? Looking at the left side of the figure, we see that (alas) even when the help source is a spouse, those who sought help from another person had slightly *higher* depression scores than those who did not (although this difference was not statistically significant). In other words, *seeking help from a spouse need not be harmful to your mental health; it just doesn't make it any better.* The right side of the figure tells a very different story regarding help from a stranger. Those who sought help there were far more depressed at Wave 3 than those who did not; this was a statistically significant difference.

There is one obvious objection to the evidence from Figure 9.1: We have failed to control for other variables that might influence the relationship. It is critical to control statistically for the worker's earlier level of distress before the helpseeking happened, and it is also important to take into account the workers' personal characteristics.

Therefore, all results for seeking help, including the professional help to which we turn next, were checked using a more complex statistical model that takes into account workers' personal characteristics, their employment status, and their previous levels of distress. In interpreting these tables, it is important to remember that including a worker's previous distress level in any equation means that the results that are observed refer to change in distress. In all cases, these analyses show that what the figures show about the differences in Wave 3 depression is also true for change in depression.

Professional Help

We also explored the issue of seeking help from a professional source. We asked workers whether they had sought the help of any of the following:

clergy, minister, priest, rabbi
marriage counselor
mental health professional (psychiatrist, psychologist, psychoanalyst)
medical doctor
social worker
"other" professional

There is an extensive literature concerning whether mental health professionals actually help, as well as whether there are differences among them in the effectiveness of treatment. We briefly review this literature next, to get a sense of what is normally to be expected from getting help of this type.

In general, studies show that psychotherapy has positive effects. Many patients who seek treatment report improved mental health (Smith, Glass, & Miller 1980). However, a small proportion of patients deteriorate after undergoing therapy (Bergin, 1971; Lambert, Shapiro, & Bergin, 1986; Smith et al., 1980). Reviews of outcome studies show that the proportion is generally in the range of 6 to 12% (Lambert et al., 1986), a figure that is remarkably consistent across a variety of studies.

There is disagreement concerning how outcomes should be assessed (Lambert, 1983; Mirin et al., 1991). It is agreed, however, that one of the important goals of psychotherapy should be the alleviation of clinical symptomatology (Mirin et al., 1991), and several factors have been shown to influence the alleviation of symptoms as a psychotherapeutic outcome. Specifically, outcomes have been shown to be linked to factors related to the therapist, factors related to the client, and factors related to the therapeutic encounter. Therapist factors commonly refer to therapist personality style or therapeutic training. Negative outcomes are often attributed to therapists who are emotionally distant or cold or who lack the skills to treat a client with a particular problem. Client factors include motivation and desire to obtain treatment and to continue treatment once begun, client personality factors, and sociodemographic factors. Finally, therapist and client may simply be unsuited for each other. They may be unable to establish the good working relationship necessary for improving the life of the client. (See Mirin et al., 1991, for a fuller discussion of these issues.)

In assessing what our plant closing study can contribute to this literature, it is important to emphasize that we do not have information on either the therapist or the therapeutic encounter. We do, however, have extensive information on the clients—the workers themselves—and therefore we look at the impact of their personal characteristics in some detail. We begin by looking at symptoms of depression and anxiety and conclude this section with a discussion of the role that self–blame may play.

Figure 9.2 shows the difference between workers who do and do not seek professional help. Again we provide several examples to show that all kinds of professional help are not equal. The figure first shows Wave 3 depression among those who did, or did not, seek help from a religious professional (clergy, minister, priest, or rabbi). This is followed by the numbers for a regular medical doctor and for a mental health professional (psychiatrist, psychologist, or psychoanalyst).

A simple glance at Fig. 9.2 tells us that if the worker sought professional help between Wave 2 and Wave 3, depression was higher than if the worker did not.

In Table 9.1, we show these results for both depression and anxiety. Again, our

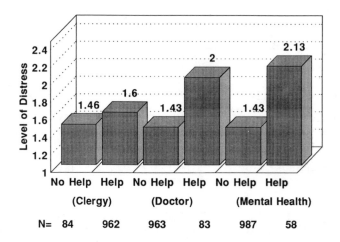

Figure 9.2. Wave 3 depression as related to seeking professional help in the preceding year.

more elaborate statistical tests showed that this conclusion for the absolute level of depression at Wave 3 was also true for *change* in depression (that is, when we controlled for Wave 2 depression scores), and it held when we took into account workers' personal characteristics and employment or unemployment (see Table 9.1). Furthermore, the other forms of professional help that were asked about but are not shown here tend to fall in between the extremes we have depicted, both in the frequency with which help was sought and its apparent impact.

So far, what we have is a striking finding, but no proof that the linkage is one of cause and effect, let alone any explanation of why the cause would cause the effect. What we have is just a fact: it may be true that all but 6 or 12% of people who see mental health professionals get better, as the scientific literature tells us, but these autoworkers were in that unhappy group who are not helped by the encounter. We next ask whether any particular groups of these workers fared better or worse when they sought professional help.

Victims of Help?

Earlier chapters had a great deal to say about the small and large personal differences in resources and life chances that can affect mental health. Therefore, it is important that we take a harder look at these personal characteristics as we ask

Table 9.1

Regression of Wave 3 Mental Health on the Use of Services Since Wave 2 [a]

Effects on	Use of Any Professional	
	Depression	Anxiety
Race (B) (1=black)	−.044	−.040
Gender (F) (1=female)	−.021	.028
Age (A)	.002	.002
Education (E)	.000	−.009
Income (I)	−.002	−.002[b]
Employed at Wave 2	.050	.055
Mental health at Wave 2	.404[c]	.476[c]
Total events excluding Financial (T3–T2)	.087[c]	.029[b]
Financial hardship (T3–T2)	.003[c]	.002[c]
Services use (T3–T2)	.149[c]	.165[c]
Constant	.576	.532
R^2	.41	.39

[a] N = 1,083. Unstandardized coefficients are presented. Workers' personal characteristics are measured as of Wave 1. Services use refers to the use of professional services measured at Wave 3 concerning the period between Wave 2 and Wave 3.
[b] $p < .05$.
[c] $p < .01$.

an ironic question: *Who appears to be most harmed (or not helped) by professional help?*

We approached this issue with a suspicion about what we might find. In the long history of debates about who benefits from therapy, there have been suggestions that perhaps mental health therapy in general, but certainly some specific therapies like psychotherapy, may be ill–suited to some patients. As Sigmund Freud rather bluntly put it,

> One should look beyond the patient's illness and form an estimate of his whole personality; those patients who do not possess a reasonable degree of education and a fairly reliable character should be refused. It must not be forgotten that there are healthy people as well as unhealthy ones who are good for nothing in life, and that there is a temptation to ascribe to their illness everything that incapacitates them if they show any sign of neurosis. (Freud, 1905/1974).

This suggests that perhaps those personal characteristics that are tied to economic resources might differentiate the response to professional help. In particular, workers who are less educated, black, or low income might fare especially badly in the hands of a mental health professional.

Therefore we next ask whether any particular worker characteristics interact with seeking help from a professional. We focus on mental health professionals as the helpers and depression as the outcome.

Figure 9.3 shows what happened to depression symptoms and to whom,

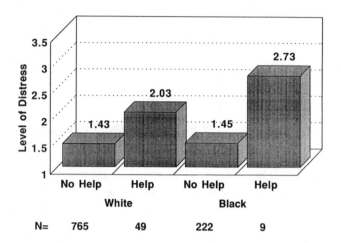

Figure 9.3a. Wave 3 depression, seeing a mental health professional, and workers' race.

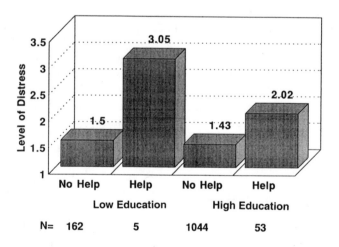

Figure 9.3b. Wave 3 depression, seeing a mental health professional, and workers' education.

subdivided first by race and second by education. Because comparisons can be very fragile when small numbers of people are involved, again we present the number of workers in each category at the bottom of the figure as a reminder.

The figures tell the story of two significant interactive effects, presented visually. There were bigger negative effects of seeing a mental health professional among blacks than among whites and among less educated workers than among those who had completed high school. Again this was true not just of the absolute level of depression at Wave 3, but also of the change in depression since Wave 2.

Explanatory Mechanisms: Self–Blame

What are we to make of these results? The lack of information on what occurred in the therapeutic encounter is a serious impediment to interpreting them. However, we were able to take a further step by focusing on self–blame. If the extent to which workers blame themselves (or the extent to which their self–blame grows over time) is a key to explaining the impact of professional services use, particularly for depression, this would support the arguments of cognitive theories that give an important role to self–blame in the genesis or maintenance of depression (Chapter Eight; see also Abramson et al., 1978; Beck, 1967, 1987). Self–blame may offer a kind of indirect window into the therapeutic encounter.

In assessing the role of self–blame, first we treated it as a dependent variable, looking at how it is linked to seeking help from a mental health professional.

Table 9.2 shows this analysis. Just as was true of anxiety and depression, seeking help between Wave 2 and Wave 3 was associated with greater self–blaming at Wave 3. We also asked, next, whether this growth in self–blame accounts for the negative association between mental health and the use of mental health professional services.

Table 9.3 reports this detailed analysis, in which we added self–blame at Wave 3 and change in self–blame since Wave 2 to the basic results from before. The impact of professional help on change in depression was largely accounted for when self–blame was controlled. This means that now growth of self–blame, an issue which we have encountered throughout the book, but most systematically in Chapter Eight, is a candidate for explaining how it is that professional "help" hurts mental health. According to this argument, it hurts by leading workers to blame themselves for their plight.

Seeking Help: What Did It Mean?

Now, it is important to take stock of whether we have really found that professional "help" *caused* a deterioration in mental health, and if so, what the mechanisms might be.

Table 9.2
Self–Blame (T3) as a Function of the Use of Services (T3–T2) [a]

	Any Professional
Race (1=black)	−.196[b]
Sex (1=female)	−.126
Age (T1)	.000
Education (T1)	−.021
Income (T1)	−.001
Employed (T2)	.097
Depression (T2)	.018
Anxiety (T2)	.276[b]
Self–blame (T2)	.191[b]
Total events excluding financial (T3–T2)	.062[b]
Financial hardship (T3–T2)	.005[b]
Services use (T3–T2)	.338[b]
Constant	.641
R^2	.26

[a] N = 1,082. Unstandardized coefficients are presented. Workers' personal characteristics are measured as of Wave 1. Services use refers to the use of professional services measured at Wave 3 concerning the period between Wave 2 and Wave 3.
[b] $p < .01$

Is the Effect Real? Self–Selection. People who had professional help for their mental troubles at one point in our study were worse off at a later point. If this does not prove that the professional encounter caused the deterioration, what did? A first

Table 9.3
Regression of Mental Health (T3) on the Use of Services (T3–T2) and Self–Blame [a]

	Use of Any Professional	
	Depression	Anxiety
Prior mental health (T2)	.335[c]	.421[c]
Total events excluding financial (T3–T2)	.069[c]	.017
Financial hardship (T3–T2)	.002[c]	.001[b]
Services use (T3–T2)	.045	.096[c]
Self–blame (T2)	.250[c]	.161[c]
Change in self–blame (T3–T2)	.301[c]	.209[c]
Constant	.367	.407
R^2	.57	.48

[a] N = 1,068. Services use refers to the use of professional services measured at Wave 3 concerning the period between Wave 2 and Wave 3. The unstandardized coefficients presented are net of race, sex, age, education, family income, and employment status.
[b] $p < .05$.
[c] $p < .01$.

consideration is the self–selection that takes place when people use professional services. This argument says that some people became worse basically because they were worse off to start with—otherwise, they wouldn't have sought help.

It is almost certainly the case that people who use professional services for mental health problems are significantly different in many ways from those who do not. The relative rarity of the use of mental health services is itself evidence of the fact that people who use services are atypical. Most studies show clearly that services users have greater levels of psychological distress; it is almost a truism to say that this is the case. Other characteristics are also likely to be associated with the use of services. Our preliminary analysis shows that people who use services have initially higher levels of self–blame, higher distress levels, and more previous utilization of mental health services. People who used mental health services also had a greater level of negative life events. The fact that such people feel bad, or have bad things happen to them, is why they seek the help of the mental health professional. This makes sense.

The threat to the validity of our results comes about if we have been unable to control for these prior differences. To the extent that our results concerning poorer mental health are change scores, we are able to say with some confidence that even though people who went to see the mental health professional were more initially distressed and self–blaming than those who did not go, *they were even more distressed and self–blaming after they used mental health services.* That is, true deterioration in mental health and an increase in self–blame result from the use of mental health services.

At some level, self–selection always remains a possible explanation of a finding such as our own. For example, it could reasonably be argued that a checklist measure is inadequate for distinguishing, and hence controlling for, true psychopathology (Coyne & Downey, 1991). But we believe that self–selection is an unsatisfactory explanation for yet another reason. A self–selection argument should not, itself, be made selectively; self–selection into therapy logically applies to the 88 to 94% of cases in which therapy helps clients as much as to the 6 to 12% of cases in which it does not (see Lambert et al., 1986).

Is the Effect Inevitable? Logically resembling the self–selection argument is the claim that entering into a relationship as a client has certain negative effects on self–concept. That is, the client must take the step of defining self as needing help and of ceding some amount of control over personal wellness to another person.

However reasonable this argument, it has the same logical status as the previous one. Defining the self as needing help and ceding control over that help occur in the overwhelming majority of successful therapeutic encounters as well as in the minority—such as those encountered here—where the client emerges more scarred. Self–labeling and loss of a sense of control may be contributing factors, just as self–selection may play a role, but it is unlikely that they fully account for the results observed.

Dynamics of Deterioration. It is possible that the results reported here are specific to affective disorders—although if so, it is still the case that our findings are relevant to a large segment of mental health problems. Because we have focused on depression and anxiety, two of the most common mental health complaints, it is important to take stock of whether the theoretical literature on these disorders can enlighten us about the possible mechanisms behind the deterioration tracked here.

Although people who are depressed are often anxious and vice versa, the two conditions are empirically and theoretically distinguishable. Depression may be a condition of helplessness and hopelessness, whereas anxiety may represent a condition of helplessness and uncertainty (Garber et al., 1980). This perspective rests on a version of the "learned helplessness" hypothesis, which says that central to depression is the experience of learning that what one does makes no difference for one's outcomes, that one is helpless (Seligman, 1975). In recent versions of this hypothesis, the authors have argued that (a) depressed affect does not in fact ensue unless an outcome is negative as well as uncontrollable and (b) central to the process is the person's attribution concerning why outcomes are beyond control (Abramson et al., 1978; Abramson, Garber and Seligman, 1980). A particularly pernicious combination is to see bad outcomes as caused by internal, stable, and global factors—in other words, to blame the self for what has happened.

The situation in which a client seeks the help of a therapist, but no improvement results, may serve simultaneously to engender learned helplessness and self–blame. This lack of improvement may occur because of the client, the therapist, or the interaction between the two. One factor we examined as a possible element in mental health deterioration was self–blaming. Initially, workers with and without jobs did not differ in their tendencies toward self–blame, as shown previously. The large, impersonal actor General Motors was the "who" (or what) that the workers regarded as responsible for their unemployment.

Similar to the results for anxiety and depression, we found that self–blame grew over time and that one factor associated with it was the use of professional services. When the level and growth of self–blame were subsequently taken into account, the impact of professional services on depression and anxiety was greatly reduced or insignificant.

Overall, then, the results for self–blame are consistent with the argument that the therapeutic encounter may build internal, stable, global attribution tendencies. The tendencies are negative. As a result, depression, anxiety (to the extent that helplessness is a component of anxiety), and self–blame feed on one another, and each may feed on the therapeutic encounter.

Class and the Consequences of Therapy. One obvious potential limitation to the generality of these results remains to be discussed. Class may be a hidden factor contributing to these findings—hidden because the entire sample consisted of blue–collar autoworkers. To the working–class client, psychotherapy is more likely viewed as simply "talking" and as having little intrinsic benefit (Garfield, 1986). This may be due to the multiple needs the person may have or to several practical problems for the working or lower class person. Fees for services, the costs of transportation, lost wages due to time missed from work, and the difficulty of arranging for time to use such services may be important obstacles to initial and follow–up use of mental health services. In the face of such difficulties, it may seem to the client that simply "talking" will not solve any problems. There is also evidence to suggest that the lower and working–class client is more likely to view symptoms as somatic in nature and that simply talking about inner emotional states, when problems are believed somatic, is ineffective. Studies of dropouts from psychotherapy provide suggestive evidence. The lower and working–class client is more likely to drop out of therapy (Garfield, 1986), and reasons typically given by lower SES dropouts from psychotherapy include negative attitudes toward therapists and treatment, as well as lack of effectiveness of psychotherapy (Garfield, 1986).

It is also possible that the lower SES client may have multiple needs when seeking the help of a therapist. It is the job of the therapist to address individual psychological problems, though clients sometimes want the therapist to address other needs. Clients may have problems of living related to their financial or job circumstances. Clients may also need someone who can intervene in the system for them – at the job placement office, the attorney's office, the welfare office, or the physician's office. Some evidence suggests that clients often are seeking more than therapy for an emotional difficulty when they engage a psychotherapist (Lorion & Felner, 1986), whereas the therapist is trained to deal only with emotional problems. Thus, divergent expectations for what can and will be accomplished in the therapeutic relationship can lead to poor outcomes. This mismatch between client and therapist goals may lead to poor outcomes. To the extent that people seek the help of a psychotherapist for something in addition to alleviation of symptoms, such as for assistance that will lead to a new job, these other needs are likely to go unaddressed. Although multiple needs may complicate any therapeutic encounter, they may be more likely when the client is economically deprived—as when, for example, an auto plant just closed.

Some of the evidence here is suggestive. Within this sample of autoworkers, more poorly educated workers who sought help from specialty sector professionals had poorer mental health, as did black workers, as did lower income workers. Perhaps these groups of workers had multiple needs and sought additional forms of assistance other than just for mental health problems. However, the lack of data on the therapeutic encounter leaves this an open question.

The bottom line in this case may be simple, although we cannot prove it yet.

It may be a matter of trust. In times of need, intimacy helps. Among the informal sources of help, a spouse is a trusted intimate, but a stranger is an unknown. Among the professional helpers, a person's minister or rabbi is a known entity and probably already trusted. But a mental health professional, to whom people do not go until things become very bad, is a stranger. And a regular medical doctor is in between—but on the basis of our data seems to be more like a stranger than a friend.

HELP IS ALL AROUND

When things go wrong in life—as they always do, for all of us, at least some of the time—other people in our lives help us to bear the burden. A large and growing body of research on the impact of such support from others has identified several forms that social support can take, and at least two ways in which any particular form of social support can affect our mental health during stressful times (see House et al., 1988).

Social support can be emotional or instrumental, and it can be individualized or collective. Emotional social support is easy to grasp: Parents love children, and friends stand by their friends in need. Instrumental social support often goes hand in hand with emotion. These same parents and friends give tangibles, like money, as well as intangibles, like love. Most of the studies of social support have focused on close ties such as these, where an individual in need is helped by other close individuals who see and are touched by this need. But when troubles are collective, it may also be important to examine the impact of organizations to which the person belongs: the union, the religious group, the local clubs. Such organizations may provide important instrumental or emotional assistance on the basis of group membership. They need not imply or require close personal ties among members, although they often engender them.

Social support from a variety of sources may generate additional, related benefits. People to whom we are tied may act to alter our behaviors, even as they provide emotional support. Some of the physical health benefits of having other people to lean on may flow from the fact that they also nag us to stop smoking, lose weight, or get a checkup. And the very flow of emotional and instrumental aid comes with activity attached. We visit and are visited by friends and relatives, we attend religious services, and we go to meetings of organizations and unions to find out how to get their help. Sources of support help to keep people busy as well as buoyed up financially or emotionally. Finally, because athletic activity can ease depression, organized athletic activity might improve mental health for both physical and social reasons.

We measured six potential sources of social support: organized athletic activity; union membership and degree of participation; membership and degree of activity in clubs and organizations; frequency of attending religious services; frequency of getting together with neighbors, friends, or relatives; and having or not having others to confide in. These questions were arranged so that the most sensitive issue, whether the person had a confidant, was asked after several items about social ties had already been answered. These questions are similar to questions asked in other studies, though we ask about issues specific to our sample (i.e., union membership) (House et al., 1988; Kessler et al., 1988).

Confidants

Exactly how does emotional social support affect mental health? There are at least two ways in which any kind of social support may be linked to mental health. Emotional support can serve as an example. First, it seems that people with support simply have better mental and physical health than people who don't. Happiness promotes health. (Of course, as noted earlier, part of the impact of loved ones may be because they inspire us to behave differently, in more health–promoting ways.) We will call this the *simple* effect of social support. Second, more subtly, people who have at least one other person to confide in and hold onto in hard times seem to be less affected by stressful experiences. This second effect of social support is called its *buffering* (or "stress buffering") role. Social support partially or fully protects the psyche from being damaged by the stress it encounters. Interestingly, buffering is the inverse of the idea, discussed earlier, that the occurrence of negative events makes a person more vulnerable to the impact of later events. Both the simple effect and the buffering effect of social support tend to be modest in size, and there has been some argument back and forth among social scientists about whether buffering, the second impact of social support, is real.

For emotional well–being the most important issue seems to be whether the person under stress has *at least one* other person to confide in. For married people, this confidant is usually the spouse, and married people are more likely than the unmarried to say "yes," there is someone around to confide in. This is likely to be part of the reason why the married, as we saw earlier, tend to be less depressed.

Earlier, we showed the first of the proposed two types of effects of social support on autoworkers' mental health. Workers who had at least one person to confide in were less depressed, regardless of their employment status. But that chapter did not ask about the buffering that social support might provide. This chapter completes the story.

Tests of the Buffering Hypothesis. The answer regarding the buffering role of social support in these data is a short: We found none. These tests were carried out by including effects of unemployment and of workers' personal characteristics and by adding to the model, at each wave, the presence/absence of a confidant and its interaction with unemployment. A final test then substituted cumulative unemployment for Wave 3 unemployment in assessing Wave 3 distress. In no case did we find a significant interaction of confidant with unemployment: Workers did not respond differently to unemployment whether they did or did not have a confidant.

Other Social Activities

A series of other questions asked about group memberships and levels of different kinds of social activity. In some cases, there was a two–step logic: First, was the worker a member? Second, how active? Our reasoning is that even a completely inactive member can potentially draw on, or activate, membership resources more readily than a nonmember. We also measured the frequency of getting together with friends and neighbors and the frequency of attending religious services. Details on the coding was presented in Chapter Two.

Union Membership: Details and Implications. In times of trouble, union membership should help for both instrumental and emotional reasons. We have already seen that to be a member of the UAW was a financially useful thing for these workers. As Chapter Three outlined, UAW membership provided workers with an array of financial benefits while they were out of work. And workers who managed to stay "within the fold" by returning to work in auto plants fared much better financially than those who moved into other manufacturing and especially into service sector jobs where the UAW no longer represented them.

Of course, union membership also has an emotional meaning. The world headquarters of the UAW is called Solidarity House for good reason. But to the extent that membership and its benefits have become a taken for granted among the modern workforce, we might expect a more instrumental than emotional tie between these workers and their union.

In the context of mental health, there is a final side to union membership that may differentiate it from other sources of social support. As a collective organization, any union offers not just a membership card but a way of looking at the world. And Chapter Eight emphasized that the worker's way of looking at the situation was crucial for understanding what aspects of mental health were affected by the plant closings, how badly, and for how long. One aspect of looking at the situation—and one ingredient in depression—is blaming the self. We have seen that workers did not tend to blame themselves for what was happening to them but that there was some tendency for self–blame to build over time. As a collective resource, the UAW potentially provided workers not only with financial assistance, but also with an ideology for understanding why plants close and who is to blame. In this context it is easy to imagine that one of the sources of the workers' widely–held view that GM was to blame—and the worker was not—may have been the UAW. The union position, as indicated in numerous press accounts, was clearly that management was at fault. (This position, of course, was a reflection of the views of the membership, as well as a potential shaper of those views.) Therefore union membership and union activism could be related to patterns of self–blame, to other elements of depression, and to anxiety.

At the outset, all workers belonged to the International Union–UAW. In both the second and third surveys, we first asked whether the worker belonged to a union, then which union, and then how often the worker attended meetings or activities. Virtually everyone (96%) who belonged to a union as of Wave 3 was a UAW member, so when we talk about the impact of "union membership" it can be understood as the impact of UAW membership, although we will use a small "u" to show that we include members of any union in these discussions.

Figure 9.4 shows just how gregarious, active, and religious these workers were at Wave 3 of the survey. We also checked for trends over the three surveys but found few except for the obvious: fewer union members at Waves 2 and 3, and the drop occurred among closing plant workers.

It is clear from this figure that membership and activity level do need to be distinguished. At one extreme, union membership is very high even at this third wave; but almost no one who is a member is very active. At another extreme, organized athletic activity is carried out by a minority of workers, and if they do it at all, they are quite regular about it. Somewhere in between stand religion and other organized clubs (which include religious ones). Finally, of the various ways of being active that we asked about, an informal one—getting together with friends and neighbors—is the most common. This is not surprising given that no membership costs or efforts are entailed, everyone has neighbors, and nearly everyone has friends.

EFFECTS OF COLLECTIVE SUPPORTS ON DEPRESSION AND SELF–BLAME

Confidants and Other Helpers

Did it matter whether workers had access to social support? To answer this question, we continue to build up our model of resources. All analyses that follow take into account the worker's personal characteristics such as race and gender. In addition, we always tested for whether the conclusions in any way depended on workers' financial hardship or the other negative life events they experienced. Then we asked whether support matters, and if so, how much and what kind.

Answering this question required making certain decisions about the way to handle the different types of support. The importance of having a confidant in other studies of social support caused us to treat it separately from the other questions about social activities. We always did two things:

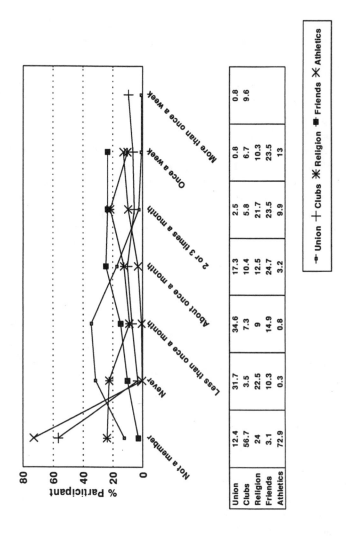

Figure 9.4. Frequency of activities.

1. In making decisions about the importance of different sources of social support for mental health, first we looked at the impact of whether or not the worker had a confidant, and then asked whether the other types of social support added to the help that is provided by a confidant. In this sense, the presence versus absence of a confidant is a kind of "first among equals" among the social support questions.

2. At the same time, the question about having a confidant is the most vulnerable to the possible criticism that what we have measured is not a cause but an effect of mental distress. If there is a linkage between lacking a confidant and being depressed, for example, who is to say that it isn't because depressed people tend to think they have no one in whom to confide (and even tend to drive away those confidants they do have)?

We could get around this problem, at least in the second and third surveys, by always using the confidant question from the previous survey. The other social support questions, in contrast, were always drawn from the same survey as the mental health outcome we were trying to predict.

These analyses treat union membership in two ways. When "union" is part of a summary measure of activities, we use all seven levels of activity that were available in the codes. But in looking at greater depth at the impact of union membership, we treat *union* as a dichotomy (union/nonunion), in the light of what Figure 9.4 shows. The key dividing line is membership, and activity adds minimal information to that.

Results

None of the types of supportive activities we have looked at added much, in and of itself, to what we know from simply asking the person if there is someone—anyone—to confide in. The largest additional factor in combating depression was provided by friends and fellow worshipers. The best medicines against self–blame were union activity and religious activity. (And both of these latter trends were very fragile.) Both unions and religions, to some extent, help to provide the worker with a world view, a way of interpreting the plant closing experience. In each case, this world view may help to move blame away from the individual worker (for example, as the situation becomes "management's fault" or "God's will").

To assess the additive effect of sources of support, we also tried combining all of the support activities—friends, athletics, clubs, union, and religion—into a single indicator. Added together, these five support activities were just about as powerful as having a confidant in predicting both depression and anxiety. Unlike a confidant—where one is enough, and more do not provide additional mental health help—supportive activities seem to provide a boost that follows the rule of "the more the better."

Interactive Supports: Union and Confidant

Of course, social support activities might act together to affect mental health. They could interact in some way. We did not test out all of the possible ways in which different forms of social support might interact with one another. The number of combinations is vast, and most would have little theoretical or practical meaning. We did, however, explore the combined impact of two key factors: having or not having a confidant and being or not being in a union. In doing so, we found that having a confidant, being a union member, and being employed or unemployed had a complex, interlocking effect on depression—and self–blame.

Figures 9.5a and 9.5b show the patterns for depression at Wave 3, first for workers who are employed and then for unemployed workers. Again we show the number of workers in each group at the bottom of each figure. When workers have jobs, we see that there is an impact of social support (confidant); but having a confidant has an effect only for nonmembers of a union. In contrast, when workers are unemployed, there is a flattening of the effects of anything else. (The patterns shown in Figure 9.5b are not statistically significant.)

Why should a confidant matter for the mental health of nonunion employed workers when it does not matter for union members? The issue could be a matter of money. Whether union members did or did not report having a confidant, they were making much more per hour than nonunion workers (more than $14 versus about $9). The issue may, therefore, be a crass matter of dollars and cents: a "confidant" is usually a spouse, and a spouse is often bringing in a paycheck. That paycheck matters more when a worker's own income is lower. Alternatively, we could be more emotionally oriented in explaining the difference. For example, union membership may itself be a kind of buffer that makes the confidant relationship less necessary. We probably cannot choose between these, but it is not necessary to do so.

Patterns of self–blaming offer another clue. Figures 9.6a and 9.6b show the patterns for self–blame across these same groups. Again, employment patterns and union membership and social support have complex and interdependent effects. First, of course, the story looks different for the employed versus the unemployed. Among employed workers, Figure 9.6a shows a big impact of having versus not having a confidant on the self–blame of the nonmember. This simply mirrors what we have already seen regarding depression. It also shows a large overall difference between union members and nonmembers. *Union members are less self–blaming.* Among unemployed workers, as was the case for depression, the differences flatten out. (The differences in Figure 9.6b are not statistically significant.)

In combination, these trends suggest to us that union membership brought advantages that were both monetary and ideological. The union member had financial advantages and cushions that the nonmember lacked, and was exposed to a way of looking at the situation—nonself–blaming—that was likely to yield mental

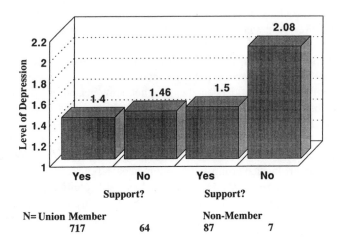

Figure 9.5a. Union membership, social support (at Wave 2), and wave 3 depression: Employed workers.

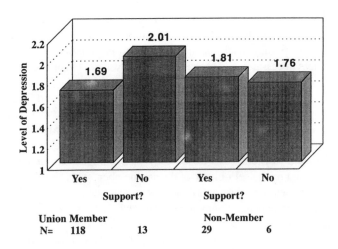

Figure 9.5b. Union membership, support (at Wave 2), and Wave 3 depression: unemployed workers.

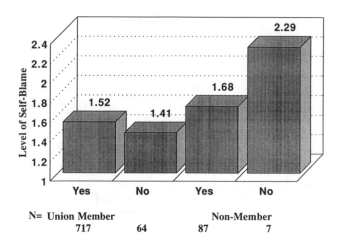

Figure 9.6a. Union membership, social support (at Wave 2), and Wave 3 self–blame : employed workers.

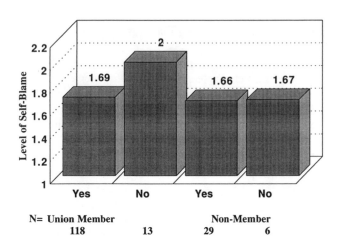

Figure 9.6b. Union membership, social support (at Wave 2), and Wave 3 depression: unemployed workers.

health benefits in these circumstances.

CONCLUSIONS

The Paradox of Help

Humans thrive when we have others we can count on, others to whom we can turn for help. As this chapter has documented, however, actually *asking* for this help does not always turn out so well. There is a sense in which social support is support as long as it is not asked for.

The chapter has already discussed the impact—largely negative—that was evident when workers as individuals sought help from other individuals. The least damage in those "helping" encounters was registered when it came from a spouse; the most, when it came from a sheer stranger or a mental health professional. We speculated about the origins of these negative trends, and located at least part of their source in the growth of self–blame. We also speculated about the possibility that the findings at least partly reflect the population under the microscope, blue–collar workers, autoworkers.

What we have here is not proof, but it is cause for concern. If these kinds of effects are particularly acute in the blue–collar segment of the population, this could have serious policy implications in an era of plant closings and blue–collar job dislocations.

Some Implications of the Helpseeking Findings

It is important to put seeking help and having ties in the context of what loss of ties does to people. Earlier chapters have shown that "negative life events" have a potent impact on mental health. These events include, of course, breaking off love relationships and the loss of loved ones through death, the loss of health through illness or accident, and the loss of peace of mind that comes from being the victim of crime. Finally, in a study like this, they include the loss of financial security that flowed from the closing of the auto plants.

In contrast to the powerful impact of negative life events, all of our analyses—including this chapter's comparisons among kinds of support—have shown that things that help, help relatively more weakly. It appears to be easier to show how mental health is harmed than how it is bolstered. Is this because we are looking at the wrong things? We do not think so. Workers probably are not as capable of telling us about how they are helped as about how they are harmed, because they do not themselves realize the extent or even the sources of help. Human beings are physically and psychologically organized to notice change. Just as we notice when a light is turned off and pay no attention to the fact that the lights are still on, so we notice that a loved one has left us and take for granted the loved one who stands by our side. Therefore this study is able to trace workers' sources of help—their loved ones and friends and God and union—but it should be expected that the picture of help will be fuzzier than the picture of harm. And it was.

Implications of the Collective Supports

What we take for granted is really a kind of everyday miracle—social support. It occurs most naturally, with least pain, in the naturally occurring groupings of family life and neighborhood, in the communities of God and common interest formed by religion and by other organizations, and in unions. For these workers, their union membership was seemingly an instrumental thing. They were union members, but their actions hardly reflected it. Most carried the card, but missed the meetings. Still, on top of the aid provided by supportive others, union membership brought two pieces of assistance, two very different types of reason to believe.

Unions gave the workers dollars. Because nearly all the union members were still UAW members as of the end of our study, we can put it this way: When they were working, UAW members made much more money per hour than nonmembers. And the workers, of course, knew that.

Unions—the UAW—also gave the workers a way of looking at their lives and at what had gone wrong with them. The UAW offered workers a reason to believe in themselves by giving them a world view that told them that what had happened was not their fault. This was one of the critical pieces of mental health for these workers.

10
Conclusions: What Have We Learned

This book set out to do two things: first, to attempt to understand the men and women who lost their jobs when General Motors closed auto plants in the late 1980's. What did downsizing mean to them and their families? Second, we wanted to understand more about the stress process.

WHAT WE FOUND

What did we find in this study? Chapter Three showed that expectations and reality were significantly linked for these workers. Workers expected little after the plant closing, and they got what they expected. Most thought it would be difficult or impossible to get a job with as good pay and benefits as the GM job, and they were correct. The new jobs that they got paid less and had poorer benefits.

We also documented how the characteristics of workers influenced the link between expectations and reality. We expected that the older, white, and male workers would begin with more resources and would be more likely to keep their jobs. This expectation was borne out. Closing plant workers were disproportionately young, black, and female. Thus, the workers who were older, white, and male, could expect and get more even though plants were closing and jobs were being lost.

In Chapter Four, we first addressed the issue of the relationship between depression and unemployment over time. Reemployment was affected through three mechanisms: (1) by being unemployed at Wave 1, (2) by being in a closing plant and not yet unemployed at Wave 1, and (3) by being depressed at Wave 1. Thus, depression which resulted from job loss also played some role in preventing workers from becoming reemployed. We further examined family conflict in

211

response to unemployment. We found evidence that unemployment leads to financial hardship and that financial hardship is the critical factor in family conflict and stress. There is a steady toll that financial hardship takes on family harmony. Further, we found that the fear of hardship had negative effects on workers whose plants did not close. Over time, broken ties and tension and strain with spouse and children generally remained the same or dropped in the closing plants. In contrast, nonclosing plant workers did less breaking up with spouses and lovers around the middle of our study, during the year after the closing of the plants, but their levels of conflict began to rise and stayed high. Therefore, although we showed how plant closings are bad for families, the fear and anticipation of job loss may also wreak silent damage even among those who have not yet lost their jobs.

In Chapter Five, we considered the issue of the workers' characteristics in the unemployment and mental health equation. What emerged in that chapter is a clear sense of differential vulnerability to unemployment among workers, depending on their demographic characteristics. Race and education played a critical role in this pattern of differential vulnerability. Education altered the impact of unemployment on distress. Unemployment had more severe effects on mental health among less educated workers. Also, throughout the study, race further modified the effect of education. Among the unemployed, black workers were particularly sensitive to educational levels. Less educated black workers were the most highly distressed, and more educated black workers were not appreciably distressed.

We argued for a kind of human capital model of workers' resources for combating stress, wherein factors such as race, income, and education affected the calculus of the meaning of unemployment. Particularly, race and education not only affect workers' overall levels of distress, but also affect the *psychological impact of an economic stressor such as unemployment.* Another way of stating the fact is that for some, unemployment is a different, more stressful event, than it is for others. We showed that this was true for people who were black (as opposed to white) and relatively poorly educated.

We also explored gender and its role in the unemployment process. At both the beginning and the end of the panel study, gender interacted with marital status (Wave 1) or accumulated unemployment (Wave 3) to generate distress. Theoretically, we argued that these effects are part of a general complex of effects of gender, marital status, and unemployment in combination and that the impact of unemployment on various gender–marital status combinations is a function of the meaning to these workers of the roles they play. In particular, we noted that the biggest effect of unemployment is observed among married males, a finding which is consistent with their potentially holding a provider role in their families. Being a male, which usually is associated with lower levels of depression and anxiety, can become a liability insofar as one of its key aspects–the subrole of "provider"–ceases to be fulfilled during a period of unemployment. Gender carries symbolic baggage, as well as economic implications.

We also noted that men and women were generally similar in their reactions to unemployment. These results–a pattern of subtle but significant trends that suggest the operation of gender roles–may be exactly what researchers should expect *when the comparison between men and women is made within class, within occupation, and within condition of current employment.* In contrast, to compare distress for employed males with distress for either housewives or females who work in quite different jobs is to load the dice in favor of finding "gender" effects.

In Chapter Six, the issue of financial hardship was addressed. We showed that closing plant workers were in consistently greater financial difficulty than nonclosing plant workers, and some of their hardships grew over time. This was to be expected, because financial hardship is known to be the central feature of job loss. Over the course of the study, we observed a systematic relationship between the number of times a worker was out of work and the financial hardships experienced. Only the steadily employed escaped financial threat. Financial hardship was also implicated as an important mechanism in generating mental distress.

Therefore, financial hardships played a multifaceted role in stress as experienced by the unemployed: (1) hardships differentiated workers such that those in greater initial hardship were more likely to experience unemployment; (2) hardships grew over time in response to unemployment; and (3) hardships served as the intervening variable through which unemployment was associated with distress.

Financial hardship also played a role in self–esteem and mastery. Each of these constructs was interwoven throughout the texture of the relationships among unemployment, financial hardship, and distress. Unemployment led to depression through the following paths:
Unemployment leads to financial hardship.
Financial hardship leads to loss of mastery.
Financial hardship leads to loss of self–esteem.
Loss of mastery leads to loss of self–esteem.
Financial hardship, low mastery, and lack of self–esteem lead to distress.
Finally, unemployment sometimes made its own unique contribution to distress.

Chapter Seven dealt with the issue of life events, both in the recent and the distant past. In this chapter, we considered the issue of "carryover" stress, because we had information on the military service experience of these workers. Significantly, combat had remarkably persistent effects. Because our data were gathered in 1989, before the Gulf War, the effects of combat referred, for the most part, to events that occurred somewhere between D–day and the fall of Saigon. But although these were old battles, they were fresh in the minds of these men when they told us about their sense of self–esteem or their feelings of depression. From our perspective, there is a permanent impact of certain identity–defining roles on the unfolding life course. Looked at from a life course perspective, each experience is a piece of the tapestry that is woven to build our lives. We all simultaneously suffer and benefit from what has gone before in life. In the case of these workers, the experience of combat was a thread that was particularly salient when they faced other crises in life. As we noted, combinations of time, place, stressors, and personal history make each individual's journey through hard times a unique one.

Chapter Eight considered the issue of psychological reactions and coping. We argued that psychological resources for combating depression included how workers decided to cope with the job situation and how they laid blame for their predicament. We showed how essential it is to take the worker's point of view into account. If they got what they wanted, they were much better off. Therefore, understanding what they wanted was critical to understanding why some workers suffered less distress than did others. We found that depression improved noticeably for

workers who wanted jobs and got them,

workers who *didn't* want jobs and *didn't* get them, and for

workers who *didn't* like their jobs and lost them.

Workers were able to take some kind of control over their situations by defining the situation in a way that worked for them. Depression receded when there was a fit between what the worker thought was happening and what did happen, *whatever that was.*

That chapter also discussed the issue of self–blame. We found that the depression associated with plant closing is special in certain ways. Workers start out not blaming themselves in the slightest, but their self–blame grows over time. It grows when they have *failed* to exert control over their fates by being unable to find jobs or by finding an inadequate job. The best way for the worker to pick up the pieces of a shattered work life is to find a new job. But trying — making efforts to get or keep a new job — can bring on self–blame when efforts fall short.

The issue of informal and professional resources for help was the topic of Chapter Nine. That chapter documented how actually asking for this help does not always turn out to be beneficial for people. The impact of seeking help was largely negative. The least damage in those "helping" encounters was registered when it came from a spouse; the most, when it came from a sheer stranger or a mental health professional. We saw that one of the factors in this negative impact of seeking help was in its effect on the growth of self–blame. Recall that workers began the study largely free of self–blame for their job loss. Those who sought help, particularly professional help, grew more self–blaming as a result.

Other forms of social support were also considered in that chapter. One was union membership. Workers derived two critical benefits from their union membership. First, was the money. Contractual guarantees for UAW members meant that the workers received up to 90% of their prelayoff pay. However, the union also gave the workers a way of looking at their lives and at what had gone wrong with them. The UAW offered workers a reason to believe in themselves by giving them a world view that told them that what had happened was not their fault. This was a critical factor in mental health for these workers.

The Stress Process

First and foremost, it was our intent to say something about the mental health consequences of the stress process, about how the minds of humans whose bodies have fallen victim to "stress" often suffer. We also tried to indicate ways in which the phenomenon of unemployment was better, worse, or simply different from other modern stressors. More specifically, we attempted to show how the unemployment that flows from industrial plant closing and corporate downsizing may differ from other joblessness.

A critical feature of our study has been that although the effects of unemployment can be devastating for individuals and their families, over time the stress of unemployment usually passes, one way or another. Workers recover, to one degree or another. Who becomes whole again and how fast are, of course, the critical questions under these circumstances. Worker's characteristics — their gender, their race, and even the amount of money they had in the bank, played an important role in differentiating how quickly stress passed and how complete the recovery was. But, all in all, these workers were a resilient bunch — a group of people who learned to handle stress if they did not already know. Recent research on resilience and thriving has been grappling with the issue of how some people survive and even thrive in the face of negative life circumstances (Carver, 1998). Given the commonality of being out of work due to temporary layoffs, strikes and plant shifts in the auto industry, these workers may be well–positioned to thrive in the face of this event—they have learned how to make the best of what on the face of it seems like a terrible situation. As an example, a history of layoffs and recalls to work may serve to teach some workers to relax and enjoy the temporary "vacation" from work, though there is anxiety about the job recall.

Future Directions: Stress Processes

Theoretically, our empirical results suggest the utility of putting together ideas about identity relevant stressors with the work on the life course paradigm. Although the plant closing had a detrimental effect on the workers who experienced it, nonetheless it is clear that these workers were not a "blank slate" to whom a devastating event happened. They had a past and a future; they were people to whom other things had happened. Good or bad, these other things played a role in conditioning them to respond in certain ways to the stressful experience. If we can further explore the link between the past and the present, both life course research and identity theory should gain from the effort.

In our work, we have shown that there is both a "sociology" and a "social psychology" to unemployment, and that both are necessary to consider to understand fully how people experience and respond to stress. One facet of this involves who the individuals are; the other, their lifetime experiences and characteristic ways of responding. This can reflect the objective conditions a person faces, as well as that individual's subjective perceptions of what is happening and what *will* happen in the future. Therefore, this book is only a beginning. We have explored the "who" and the "when" of vulnerability to stress and some of the "why." A great deal more work remains to establish what helps bring vulnerable people out of hard times.

References

Abramson, L. Y., Garber, J., & Seligman, M. E. P. (1980). Learned helplessness in humans: An attributional analysis. In. J. Garber & M. E. P. Seligman (Eds.), *Human helplessness* (pp. 3–34). New York: Academic.

Abramson, L. Y., Metalsky, G. I., & Alloy, L. B. (1989). Hopelessness depression: A theory–based subtype. *Psychological Review, 96,* 358–372.

Abramson, L. Y., Seligman, M. E. P., & Teasdale, J. D. (1978). Learned helplessness in humans: Critique and reformulation. *Journal of Abnormal Psychology, 87,* 49–74.

Appy, Christian G. (1993). *Working-class war: American combat soldiers and Vietnam.* Chapel Hill: University of North Carolina Press.

Bandura, A. (1977). Self–efficacy: Toward a unifying theory of behavioral change. *American Psychologist, 37,* 122–147.

Bandura, A. (1986). *Social foundations of thought and action: A social cognitive theory.* Englewood Cliffs, NJ: Prentice–Hall.

Bandura, A. (1995). *Self-efficacy in changing societies.* Cambridge: Cambridge University Press.

Beck, A. T. (1967). *Depression: Clinical, experimental, and theoretical aspects.* New York: Hoeber.

Beck, A. T. (1976). *Cognitive therapy and the emotional disorders.* New York: International Universities Press.

Beck, A. T. (1987). Cognitive models of depression. *Journal of Cognitive Psychotherapy, 1,* 5–37.

Beck, A. T., Rush, A. J., Shaw, B, F., & Emery, G. (1979). *Cognitive therapy of depression.* New York: Guilford Press.

Bergin, A. E. (1971). The evaluation of therapeutic outcomes. In A. E. Bergin & S. L. Garfield (Eds.), *Handbook of psychotherapy and behavioral change: An empirical analysis* (pp. 217–270). New York: Wiley.

Bluestone, B., & Harrison, B. (1982). *The deindustrialization of America.* New York: Basic Books.

Bordieu, P. (1986). The forms of capital. In J. G. Richardson (Ed.), *Handbook of theory and research in the sociology of education.* New York: Greenwood Press.

Boulanger, G., & Kadushin, C. (1986). *The Vietnam veteran redefined: Fact and fiction.* Hillsdale, NJ: Lawrence Erlbaum.

Brod, H. (1992). *The making of masculinities: The new men's studies.* New York: Routledge.

Broman, C .L., Hamilton, V. L., & Hoffman, W. S. (1990). Unemployment and its effect on families: Evidence from a plant closing study. *American Journal of Community Psychology, 18,* 643–659.

Broman, C. L.,. Jackson, J. S., & Neighbors, H. W. (1989). Sociocultural context and racial group identification among black adults. *Revue Internationale de Psychologie Sociale, 2,* 369–379.

Brown, G. W. & Harris, T. (1978). *Social origins of depression.* London, England: Tavistock.

Burke, P. J. (1991). Identity processes and social stress. *American Sociological Review, 56,* 836–849.

Burke, P. J., & Reitzes, D. C. (1981). The link between identity and role performance. *Social Psychology Quarterly, 44,* 83-92.

Burke, P. J., & Reitzes, D. C. (1991). An identity theory approach to commitment. *Social Psychology Quarterly, 54,* 239-251.

Buss, T. F., & Redburn, F. S. (1983). *Mass unemployment and community mental health.* Beverly

Hills, CA: Sage.

Calvin, D. A., Hamilton, V. L., Broman, C. L., & Hoffman, W. S. (1996). War, work, and wedlock in blue collar lives: Stressful experiences and enduring distress. Unpublished manuscript.

Campbell, D. M. (1984). *Women at war with America: Private lives in a patriotic era.* Cambridge, MA: Harvard University Press.

Caplan, R. D., Vinokur, A. D., Price, R. H., & Van Ryn, M. (1989). Job seeking, reemployment, and mental health: A randomized field experiment in coping with job loss. *Journal of Applied Psychology, 74,* 759–769.

Card, J. J. (1983). *Lives after Vietnam: The personal impact of military service.* Lexington, MA: Lexington Books.

Carver, C. S. (1998). Resilience and thriving: Issues, models, and linkages. *Journal of Social Issues, 54, 245–266.*

Cassel, J. (1976). The contribution of the social environment to host resistance. *American Journal of Epidemiology, 102,* 107–123.

Cobb, S., & Kasl, S. V. (1977). *Termination: The consequences of job loss.* Cincinnati: Department of Health Education and Welfare (NIOSH).

Cook, T. D., & Campbell, D. T. (1979). *Quasi–experimentation: Design and analysis issues for field settings.* Boston: Houghton Mifflin.

Coyne, J. C. (1992). Cognition in depression: A paradigm in crisis. *Psychological Inquiry, 3,* 232–235.

Coyne, J. C., & Downey, G. (1991). Social factors and psychopathology: Stress, social support, and coping processes. *Annual Review of Psychology, 42,* 401–425.

Coyne, J. C. & Lazarus, R. S. (1980). Cognitive style, stress perception, and coping. In I. L. Kutash & L. B. Schlesinger (Eds.), *Handbook on stress and anxiety: Contemporary knowledge, theory, and treatment* (pp. 144–158). San Francisco: Jossey–Bass.

Derogatis, L. R., Lipman, R. S., Rickels, K., Uhlenhuth, E. H., & Covi, L. (1974). The Hopkins Symptom Checklist (HSCL): A self–report symptom inventory. *Behavioral Science, 19,* 1–15.

Dohrenwend, B. S., & Dohrenwend, B. P. (1981). Life stress and illness: Formulation of the issues. In B. S.Dohrenwend & B. P. Dohrenwend (Eds.), *Stressful life events and their contexts.* New York: Prodist.

Dohrenwend, B. S., Krasnoff, L., Askenasy, A. R., & Dohrenwend, B. P. (1978). Exemplification of a method for scaling life events: The PERI Life Events scale. *Journal of Health and Social Behavior, 19,* 205–229.

Dooley, D., & Catalano, R. A. (1988). Recent research on the psychological effects of unemployment. *Journal of Social Issues, 44,* 1–12.

Dudley, K. (1994). *The end of the line: Lost jobs, new lives in postindustrial America.* Chicago: University of Chicago Press.

Elder, G. H., Jr. (1974). *Children of the Great Depression: Social change in life experience.* Chicago: The University of Chicago Press.

Elder, G. H., Jr. (1985). *Life course dynamics: Trajectories and transitions 1968-1980.* Ithaca, NY: Cornell University.

Elder, G. H., Jr. (1986). Military times and turning points in men's lives. *Developmental Psychology, 22,* 233-245.

Elder, G. H., Jr. (1987). War mobilization and the Life Course: A cohort of World War II veterans. *Sociological Forum, 2,* 449-472.

Elder, G. H., Jr. (1994).Time, human agency, and social change: Perspectives on the Life Course. *Social Psychology Quarterly, 57,* 4-15.

Elder, G. H., Jr., & Clipp, E. C. (1988a). Combat experience, comradeship, and psychological health. In J. P. Wilson, Z. Harel, & B. Kahana (Eds.), *Human adaptation to extreme stress: From the Holocaust to Vietnam* (pp. 131-156). New York: Plenum.

Elder, G. H., Jr., & Clipp, E. C. (1988b). Wartime losses and social bonding: Influences across 40 years in men's lives. *Psychiatry, 51,* 177-198.

Elder, G. H., Jr., & Clipp, E. C. (1989). Combat experience and emotional health: Impairment and

Elder, G. H., Jr., & Hareven, T K. (1993). Rising above life's disadvantage: From the Great Depression to World War. In G. H. Elder, Jr., J. Modell, & R. D. Parks (Eds.), *Children of their times: Developmental and historical insights* (pp. 47-72). New York: Cambridge University Press.

Elder, G. H., Jr., & O'Rand, A. M. (1995). Adult lives in a changing society. In K. S. Cook, G. A. Fine, & J. S. House (Eds.), *Sociological perspectives on social psychology* (pp. 452-475). Needham Heights, MA: Allyn and Bacon.

Elder, G. H., Jr., Gimbel, C., & Ivie, R. (1991). Turning points in life: The case of military service and war. *Military Psychology, 3,* 215-231.

Farrell, W. (1993). *The myth of male power: Why men are the disposable sex.* New York: Simon & Schuster.

Feather, N. T. (1990). *The psychological impact of unemployment.* New York: Springer Verlag.

Figley, C. R., & Leventman, S. (1980). *Strangers at home: Vietnam veterans since the war.* New York: Praeger.

Fisher, J. D., & Nadler, A. (1974). The effect of similarity between donor and recipient on reactions to aid. *Journal of Applied Social Psychology, 4,* 230–243.

Fisher, J. D., Nadler, A., & Whitcher–Alagna, S. (1982). Recipient reactions to aid. *Psychological Bulletin, 91,* 27–54.

Folkman, S. (1984). Personal control and stress and coping processes: A theoretical analysis. *Journal of Personality and Social Psychology, 46,* 839–852.

Folkman, S., & Lazarus, R. S. (1980). An analysis of coping in a middle–aged community sample. *Journal of Health and Social Behavior, 21,* 219–239.

Folkman, S. & Lazarus, R. (1985). If it changes it must be a process: Study of emotion and coping during three stages of a college examination. *Journal of Personality and Social Psychology, 48,* 150–170.

Forthofer, M. S., Kessler, R. C., Story, A. L., & Gotlib, I. H. (1996). The effects of psychiatric disorders on the probability and timing of first marriage. *Journal of Health and Social Behavior, 37,* 121–132.

Freud, S. (1905/1974). On psychotherapy. In. J. Strachey, (Ed.), *The standard edition of the complete psychological works of Sigmund Freud, v. 7.* London: The Hogarth Press.

Frey-Wouters, E., & Laufer R. S. (1986). *Legacy of a war: The American soldier in Vietnam.* Armonk, NY: M. E. Sharpe.

Garber, J., Miller, S. M., & Abramson, L. Y. (1980). On the distinction between anxiety and depression: Perceived control, certainty, and probability of goal attainment. In. J. Garber & M. E. P. Seligman (Eds.), *Human helplessness* (pp. 131-169). New York: Academic Press.

Garfield, S. L. (1986). Research of client variables in psychotherapy. In S. L. Garfield & A. E. Bergin (Eds.), *Handbook of psychotherapy and behavior change* (pp. 213–256). New York: Wiley.

Gecas, V. (1989). The social psychology of self-efficacy. *Annual Review of Sociology, 8,* 1-33.

Gilbert, P. (1992). *Depression: The evolution of powerlessness.* New York: Guilford Press.

Goldberger, L., & Breznitz, S. (1982). *Handbook of stress: Theoretical and clinical aspects.* New York: Free Press.

Gove, W. R. (1972). The relationship between sex roles, marital status, and mental illness. *Social Forces, 51,* 34–44.

Haaga, D. A. F., Dyck, M. J., & Ernst, D. (1991). Empirical status of cognitive theory of depression. *Psychological Bulletin, 110,* 215–236.

Hamilton, V. L., Broman, C. L., Hoffman, W. S., & Renner, D. S. (1990). Hard times and vulnerable people: Initial effects of plant closing on autoworkers' mental health. *Journal of Health and Social Behavior, 31,* 123–140.

Hamilton, V. L., Hoffman, W. S., Broman, C. L., & Rauma, D. (1993). Unemployment, distress, and coping: A panel study of autoworkers. *Journal of Personality and Social Psychology, 65,* 234–247.

Helzer, J. E., Robins, L. N., & Davis, D. H. (1976). Depressive disorders in Vietnam returnees. *The Journal of Nervous and Mental Disease, 163,* 177-185.

Herz, D. E. (1991). Worker displacement still common in the late 1980's. *Monthly Labor Review, 114(5),* 3–9.

Hobfoll, S. E. (1988). *The ecology of stress.* Washington, D.C.: Hemisphere.

Hobfoll, S. E. (1989). Conservation of resources: A new attempt at conceptualizing stress. *American Psychologist, 44,* 513–24.

Hogan, D. P. (1981). *Transitions and social change: The early lives of American men.* New York: Academic Press.

Holmes, T. H., & Rahe, R. H. (1967). The social readjustment rating scale. *Journal of Psychosomatic Research, 11,* 213–218.

House, J. S., Umberson, D., & Landis, K. (1988). Structures and processes of social support. *Annual Review of Sociology, 14,* 293–318.

Ivie, R. L., Gimbel, C., & Elder, G. H., Jr. (1991). Military experience and attitudes in later life: Contextual influences across forty years. *Journal of Political and Military Sociology, 19,* 101-117.

Jahoda, M. (1982). *Employment and unemployment: A social–psychological analysis.* Cambridge, England: Cambridge University Press.

Jahoda, M., Lazersfeld, P. M., & Zeisel, H. (1933). *Marienthal: The sociography of an unemployed community.* Chicago: Aldine Atherton.

Janoff–Bulman, R. (1979). Characterological versus behavioral self–blame: Inquiries into depression and rape. *Journal of Personality and Social Psychology, 37,* 1798–1809.

Jones, E. E., & Nisbett, R. E. (1972). The actor and the observer: Divergent perceptions in the causes of behavior. In E. E. Jones, D. E. Kanouse, H. H. Kelley, R. E. Nisbett, S. Valins, & B. Weiner (Eds.), *Attribution: Perceiving the cause of behavior.* Morristown, NJ: General Learning Press.

Judge, G. C., Griffiths, W. E., Hill, R. C., & Lee, T. (1980). *Introduction to the theory and practice of econometrics.* New York: Wiley.

Kelvin, P., & Jarrett, J. E. (1985). *Unemployment: Its social psychological effects.* Cambridge, England: Cambridge University Press.

Kessler, R. C., & Greenberg D. F. (1981). *Linear panel analysis: Models of quantitative change.* New York: Academic Press.

Kessler, R. C., & Neighbors, H. W. (1986). A new perspective on the relationships among race, social class, and psychological distress. *Journal of Health and Social Behavior, 27,* 107–115.

Kessler, R. C., House, J. S., & Turner, J. B. (1987a). Unemployment and health in a community sample. *Journal of Health and Social Behavior, 28,* 51–59.

Kessler, R. C., Price, R. H., & Wortman, C. B. (1985). Social factors in psychopathology: Stress, social support, and coping processes. *Annual Review of Psychology, 36,* 531–72.

Kessler, R. C., Turner, J. B., & House, J. S. (1987b). Intervening processes in the relationship between unemployment and health. *Psychological Medicine, 17,* 949–961.

Kessler, R. C., Turner, J. B., & House, J. S. (1988). Effects of unemployment on health in a community survey: Main, modifying, and mediating effects. *Journal of Social Issues, 44,* 69–85.

Kessler, R. C., Turner, J. B., & House, J. S. (1989). Unemployment, reemployment, and emotional functioning in a community sample. *American Sociological Review, 54,* 648–657.

Kimmel, M. S. (1996). *Manhood in America: A cultural history.* New York: Free Press.

Lambert, M. J. (1983). Introduction to the assessment of psychotherapy outcome. In M. J. Lambert, E. R. Christensen, & S. S. DeJulio (Eds.), *The assessment of psychotherapy outcomes* (pp. 3–32). New York: Wiley.

Lambert, M. J., Shapiro, D. A., & Bergin, A. E. (1986). The effectiveness of psychotherapy. In S. L. Garfield & A. E. Bergin (Eds.), *Handbook of psychotherapy and behavior change* (pp. 157–211). New York: Wiley.

Langer, E. (1983). *The psychology of control*. Beverly Hills, CA: Sage.

Lazarus, R. S. (1966). *Psychological stress and the coping process*. New York: McGraw–Hill.

Lazarus, R. S., & Folkman, S. (1984). *Stress, appraisal, and coping*. New York: Springer Verlag.

Levy, F. (1987). *Dollars and dreams: The changing American income distribution*. New York: Norton.

Levy, F., & Michel, R. C. (1991). *The economic future of American families: Income and wealth trends*. Washington DC: The Urban Institute Press.

Liem, R., & Liem, J. H. (1988). Psychological effects of unemployment on workers and their families. *Journal of Social Issues, 44,* 87–105.

Lobo, F., & Watkins, G. (1995). Late career unemployment in the 1990s. *Journal of Family Studies, 1,* 103–113.

Lorion, R. P., & Felner, R. D. (1986). Research in mental health interventions with the disadvantaged. In S. L. Garfield & A. E. Bergin (Eds.), *Handbook of psychotherapy and behavior change* (pp. 739–775). New York: Wiley.

Milkman, R. (1997). *Farewell to the factory*. Berkeley: University of California Press.

Mirin, S. M., Gossett, J. T., & Grob, M. C. (1991). *Psychiatric treatment: Advances in outcome research*. Washington, DC: American Psychiatric Press.

Mirowsky, J., & Ross, C. E. (1990). Control or defense? Depression and the sense of control over good and bad outcomes. *Journal of Health and Social Behavior, 31,* 71–86.

Moen, P., Kain, E. L., & Elder, G. H., Jr. (1983). Economic conditions and family life: Contemporary and historical perspectives. In R. R. Nelson & F. Skidmore (Eds.), *American families and the economy: The high costs of living* (pp. 213-259). Washington, DC: National Academy Press.

Monroe, S. M., & Simons, A. D. (1991). Diathesis–stress theories in the context of life stress research: Implications for the depressive disorders. *Psychological Bulletin, 110,* 406–425.

Moskos, C. C. (1986). The American enlisted man in the all-volunteer army. In D. R. Segal & H. W. Sinaiko (Eds.), *Life in the rank and file* (pp. 35-57). McLean, VA: Pergamon-Brassey's.

Owens, T. J. (1993). Accentuate the positive – and the negative. *Social Psychology Quarterly, 56,* 288–299.

Pappas, G. (1989). *The magic city: Unemployment in a working class community*. Ithaca, NY: Cornell University Press.

Pearlin, L. I. (1989). The sociological study of stress. *Journal of Health and Social Behavior, 30,* 241–256.

Pearlin, L. I., Lieberman, M. A., Menaghan, E. G., & Mullan, J. T. (1981). The stress process. *Journal of Health and Social Behavior, 22,* 337–356.

Perrucci, R., Perrucci, C. C, Targ, D., & Targ, H. T. (1988). *Plant closings: International context and social costs*. New York: Aldine de Gruyter.

Peterson, C., Schwartz, S. M., & Seligman, M. E. P. (1981). Self–blame and depressive symptoms. *Journal of Personality and Social Psychology, 41,* 253–259.

Riley, A., & Burke, P. J. (1995). Identities and self-verification in the small group. *Social Psychology Quarterly, 58,* 61-73.

Ritter, C. (1984). Occupational stress and depression among Vietnam veterans. *Journal of Sociology and Social Welfare, 11,* 826-852.

Rodgers, W. L. (1989). Comparison of alternative approaches to the estimation of simple causal models from panel data. In D. Kasprzyk, G. J. Duncan, G. Kalton, & M. P. Singh (Eds.), *Panel surveys* (pp. 432–456). New York: Wiley.

Rosenberg, M. (1965). *Society and the adolescent self-image*. Princeton, NJ: Princeton University Press.

Rosenberg, M. (1979). *Conceiving the self*. Malabar, FL: Krieger.

Rosenberg, M. (1981). The self-concept: Social product and social force. In M. Rosenberg & R. Turner (Eds.), *Social psychology: Sociological perspectives* (pp. 593-624). New York: Basic Books.

Ross, C., & Huber, J. (1985). Hardship and depression. *Journal of Health and Social Behavior, 26,* 312–327.

Ross, C. E., Mirowsky, J., & Huber, J. (1983). Marriage patterns and depression. *American Sociological Review, 48,* 809-823.

Ryder, N. B. (1965). The cohort as a concept in the study of social change. *American Sociological Review, 30,* 843-861.

Segal, D. (1977). Illicit drug use in the U.S. Army. *Sociological Symposium (Military Sociology), 18,* 66-83.

Seligman, M. E. (1975). *Helplessness: On depression, development, and death.* San Francisco: Freeman.

Selye, H. (1956). *The stress of life.* New York: McGraw–Hill.

Selye, H. (1976). *Stress in health and disease.* Boston: Butterworth.

Severo, R., & Milford, L. (1989). *The wages of war: When America's soldiers came home--From Valley Forge to Vietnam.* New York: Simon & Schuster.

Shrout, P. E., Link, B. G., Dohrenwend, B. P., Skodol, A. E., Stueve, A., & Mirotznik, J. (1989). Characterizing life events as risk factors for depression: The role of fateful loss events. *Journal of Abnormal Psychology, 98,* 460–467.

Smith, M. L., Glass, G. V., & Miller, T. I. (1980). *The benefits of psychotherapy.* Baltimore, MD: Johns Hopkins Press.

Snyder, K. A., & Nowak, T. C. (1984). Job loss and demoralization: Do women fare better than men? *International Journal of Mental Health, 13,* 193–210.

Stouffer, S. A., Suchman, E. A., DeVinney, L. C., Star, S. A., & Williams, R. M., Jr. (1949). *The American Soldier.* Princeton, NJ: Princeton University Press.

Stryker, S. (1980). *Symbolic interactionism: A social structural version.* Palo Alto, CA: Benjamin/Cummings.

Sweeney, P. D., Anderson, K., & Bailey, S. (1986). Attributional style in depression: A meta–analytic review. *Journal of Personality and Social Psychology, 50,* 974–991.

Tennen, H., & Affleck, G. (1990). Blaming others for threatening events. *Psychological Bulletin, 108,* 209–232.

Thoits, P. A. (1983). Dimensions of life events that influence psychological distress: An evaluation and synthesis of the literature. In H. B. Kaplan (Ed.), *Psychosocial stress: Trends in theory and research* (pp. 33-103). New York: Academic Press.

Thoits, P. A. (1991). On merging identity theory and stress research. *Social Psychology Quarterly, 54,* 101–112.

Thoits, P. A. (1992). Identity structures and psychological well–being: Gender and marital status comparisons. *Social Psychology Quarterly, 55,* 236–256.

Thoits, P. A. (1995). Stress, coping, and social support processes: Where are we? What next? *Journal of Health and Social Behavior, (Extra Issue),* 53-79.

U.S. Department of Health and Human Services. Public Health Service. Centers for Disease Control. (1988). Health status of Vietnam veterans: Findings from CDC Vietnam Experience Study. *Journal of the American Medical Association, 259,* 2701-2719.

Veroff, J., Douvan, E., & Kulka, R. A. (1981). *The Inner American.* New York: Basic Books.

Vinokur, A., Caplan, R. D., & Williams, C. C. (1987). Effects of recent and past stress on mental health: Coping with unemployment among Vietnam veterans and nonveterans. *Journal of Applied Social Psychology, 17,* 708–728.

Wandersee, W. D. (1981). *Women's work and family values 1920-1940.* Cambridge, MA: Harvard University Press.

Wandersee-Bolin, W. D. (1978). The economics of middle-income family life: Working women during the great depression. *Journal of American History, 65,* 60-74.

Warr, P. B. (1987). *Work, unemployment, and mental health.* New York: Oxford University Press.

Warr, P., & Parry, G. (1982). Paid employment and women's psychological well–being. *Psychological Bulletin, 91,* 498–551.

White, L. K., Booth, A., & Edwards, J. N. (1986). Children and marital happiness: Why the negative correlation? *Journal of Family Issues, 7,* 131–147.

Index